HUMANS ARE HERBIVORES
A Scientific Case for Veganism

By Adam Riva

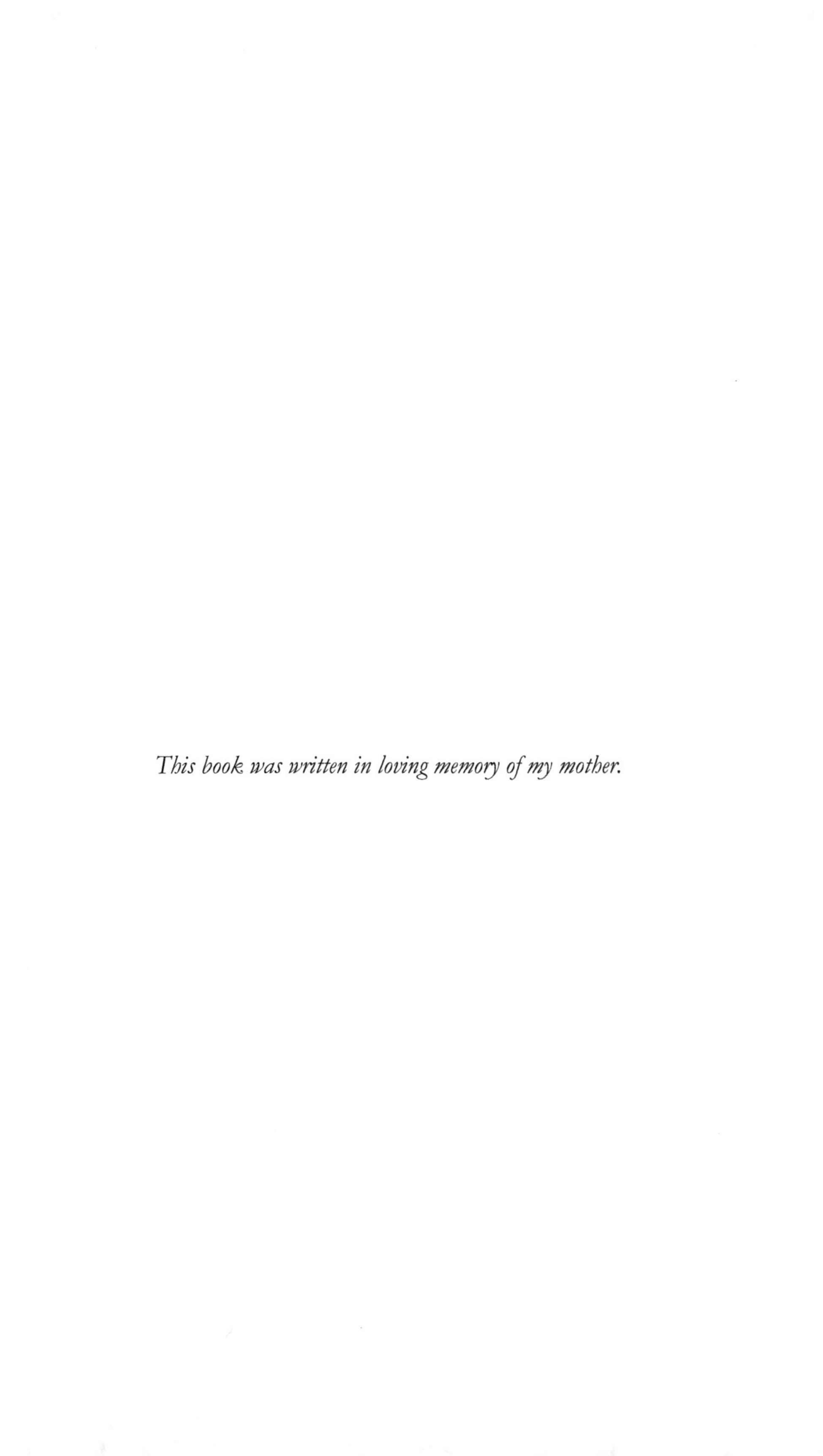

This book was written in loving memory of my mother.

CONTENTS

INTRODUCTION

Despite the abundance of medical literature readily available to ordinary people, a persistent ignorance of basic nutrition has plagued even the most health conscious eaters, even now in the 21st century. In fact, the preponderance of information has served more to confuse than to clarify.

The predicament is not as simple as people being blissfully unaware of the underlying manipulation of data and the existence of conflicts of interest. Actually, when you speak with consumers within the food industry, most people will tell you that propaganda definitely exists. However, ten different people will report ten different culprits responsible for peddling the propaganda.

So, it is not that individuals are unaware of deceptive information and junk science. The problem is that most people cannot easily navigate through the competing interests and thusly struggle to decide what they should eat and what they should avoid. Although this confusion is commonplace, the scientific community has been quite clear and consistent on its findings for at least half a century.

This book is intended to be a Magna Carta to help translate scientific jargon into plain English for those disinclined to read it and interpret it themselves. Although the data itself is nuanced, the methodologies and their conclusions are explained and sequenced to build a compelling case for eating a whole food plant-based diet.

The overall argument for veganism has four foundational pillars. The four positions are medical, anatomical, environmental, and ethical (although there is a compelling economical argument to be made, as well). Veganism often refers not only to the diet but also the lifestyle committed to avoiding animal products. The backbone of this book is science. However, I have also included the ethical argument in this book, syllogistically outlining the moral superiority of veganism for those who wish to understand it. Regardless of the morality of veganism, the medical, anatomical, and environmental arguments stand on their own.

This book is authored will the full awareness that many will attempt to discredit it simply based on the fact that it comes with moral component and is not limited to a medical or anatomical analysis. However, the philosophical proof has stood up to intellectual rigor and is equally as prudent in this discussion for the foundational reason that *ability* does not justify *morality*. Just because we *can* do something does not mean we *should*.

Do not let the author's moral stance turn you off to the underlying scientific journalism. The data and the arguments themselves should remain the focus of this book. If you are not convinced that humans are herbivores by the time you finish reading this book, then I did not do my job properly.

CHAPTER I
MEDICAL EVIDENCE DEMONSTRATING HUMANS ARE HERBIVORES

Between diet and exercise, the former is generally more divisive when it comes to right and wrong. If you're like me, you find it particularly annoying when individuals debate dietary advice without the facts. "Show me the science," is what I always say. And quite frankly, we should all demand the science and leave aside anecdotes and opinions.

All around the world, animals and their byproducts are eaten in great abundance. Most people are raised on animal products, so they never question their safety and healthfulness. With so many fad diets and conflicting theories, it can be hard to separate fact from fiction. Thankfully, the science is in, but unfortunately, most people have not seen the science for themselves, or they don't know how to interpret it. Are animal products healthy for humans? There's a simple answer, but it requires some explanation. Let's begin with some fundamentals.

Cholesterol

Animal products represent the only source of dietary cholesterol. Because of a genetic variability with cholesterol baselines, two people who follow identical diets can score differently on serum cholesterol tests. This is absolutely critical to understand when designing an experiment to study cholesterol as a dietary risk factor, and scientists have known this since 1979.[1]

Generally speaking, only one type of study is appropriate when examining the relationship between cholesterol consumption and coronary heart disease. This type of study is known as a metabolic ward study and it is the only study design capable of providing accurate results because it accounts for cholesterol baseline variability whether it is caused genetically or dietarily. Other types of study design are not applicable in this situation, such as cross-sectional population studies and other types of epidemiological studies, such as case-control or prospective cohort studies. When used to study cholesterol, these types of studies are often funded by the meat, dairy, and egg industries because they are known to generate misleading results.[2]

Prospective cohort studies are by design incapable of finding a link between cholesterol consumption and heart disease risk.[3]

It's as if you are having a foot race with your friend to see who is faster, except your friend gets a 10-yard head start. If you both finish the race at the same time, your friend might insist that he is just as fast as you. However, you know he is actually slower because you covered a greater distance in the same amount of time. The same goes for population groups that consume cholesterol; Studies need to account for the starting place.

Yet, still to this day, many researchers set up faulty studies that do not normalize cholesterol baseline levels, such as Siri-Tarino et al.'s 2010 meta-analysis which, unfortunately, many people cite all too often.[4] If you look at the references, it is funded in part by the National Dairy Council and one of the lead researchers, Ronald M. Krauss, receives funding from the meat and dairy industries.[5] This is what we call junk science and it proves the aforementioned conflicts of interest.

This is not the only example of junk science when it comes to cholesterol. For instance, if a study starts with what is called a "sick population," meaning their cholesterol scores are already sky-high, then even a study that normalizes for baseline variability can still show little or no correlation with heart disease risk. This is because cholesterol has an exponential decrease in absorption at higher levels and will form a parabolic arc when you plot the points on a graph.[6]

Often studies will observe individuals who are starting with alarmingly high cholesterol scores and then proclaim that because there was no significant change in serum levels by consuming more cholesterol, that there must not be any correlation.

Again, this is because adding cholesterol to a diet already high in cholesterol will not show any dramatic change in serum levels.[6]

By 1997, a meta-analysis of 395 metabolic ward studies by Clarke et al. concluded that dietary cholesterol has a positive correlation with serum cholesterol and coronary heart disease.[7]

Furthermore, the optimal LDL cholesterol range was reaffirmed in 2004 by O'Keefe and associates.[8] According to their study, the ideal range for low-density lipoprotein is 50-70 mg/dl, showing that there is a correlation between LDL consumption and atherosclerosis and coronary heart disease.

"No major safety concerns have surfaced in studies that lowered LDL to this range of 50 to 70 mg/dl."

This is backed up by findings from von Birgelen et al. that demonstrate a positive linear relation between LDL and coronary plaque buildup above 75mg/dL.[9] These studies properly adjusted for baseline variability, and what do you know? They conclusively demonstrated the toxicity of cholesterol.

"There is a positive linear relation between LDL cholesterol and annual changes in plaque size, with an LDL value of 75 mg/dL predicting, on average, no plaque progression."

Additionally, vegetarians put on an omnivorous diet had their cholesterol levels rise by 19%, but after only two weeks back on their original diets their cholesterol scores returned to normal.[10]

In 2006, Cohen and colleagues published a paper on the connection between low plasma-LDL levels and its protection against coronary heart disease (CHD).[11] The results were shocking and showed that even in populations with a high prevalence of cardiovascular risk factors, LDL was associated with a "substantial" increase in coronary events.

"These data indicate that moderate lifelong reduction in the plasma level of LDL cholesterol is associated with a substantial reduction in the incidence of coronary events, even in populations with a high prevalence of non—lipid-related cardiovascular risk factors."

In 2012, Ference et al. found that decreased exposure to LDL cholesterol in childhood was associated with "a substantially greater reduction in the risk of CHD."[12]

It is worth mentioning that there is a misconception that 75% of victims of heart disease fall within the "normal" range of cholesterol levels. This misconception is largely thanks to a 2009 paper by Sachdeva et al. that characterized the normal levels as anything below 130 mg/dl[13], which is 2-3 times the optimal range established by O'Keefe and associates in 2004.[8] Admittedly, only 1.4% of the patients in Sachdeva's study fell within the optimal range.

Until now, we've only discussed cholesterol as a risk factor for heart disease. In 2011, Kitahara and colleagues proved that higher total cholesterol scores were associated with several different types of cancers by examining nearly 1.2 million Korean adults for 14 years.[14]

We also have a clearly established link between cholesterol and breast cancer development, as shown in this 2012 study by Danilo and Frank.[15]

> *"…cholesterol is capable of regulating proliferation, migration, and signaling pathways in breast cancer."*

And in a 2006 paper by Li et al., it was shown that cholesterol-rich lipid rafts feed cancer cells and are associated with cellular death. It also doesn't help that dietary cholesterol promotes the oxidation of LDL cholesterol.[16]

In 2002, J.C. de la Torre published findings that Alzheimer's is partially a vascular disorder caused by lack of blood flow to the brain because of dietary cholesterol.[17]

It is crucial to remember that we are not only talking about cholesterol in meat. Remember, dairy, eggs, cheese, and other animal products also contain the cholesterol we are discussing here.

So, if cholesterol is extremely unhealthy, do we have any research demonstrating the cessation or reversal of disease after individuals cut cholesterol out of their diets? In fact, we do.

Dr. Caldwell Esselstyn has been helping patients reverse coronary heart disease with a whole foods plant-based diet for nearly 30 years. He published the bestselling book *Prevent and Reverse Heart Disease* which was based on the results of his 20-year nutritional study, the longest study of its kind ever conducted.[18]

He continues his involvement in this research to the present, with his initial results being corroborated with follow-up studies in 2007[19], 2008[20], and 2014[21], respectively.

Cholesterol is a vast subject with many nuances, controversial viewpoints, and confusion. We will analyze many of these common misconceptions in Chapter Two.

Alright, now let's talk about saturated fat.

Saturated Fat and Trans Fat

Just like cholesterol, saturated fat is predominantly found in animal products, with very few exceptions such as coconut, palm, and peanuts – but not all saturated fats are created equal. The very few exceptions of plant-based saturated fats are still much healthier by comparison because they are medium-chain triglycerides which can actually help lower LDL, burn fat, and boost metabolism.

Saturated fat raises large-particle LDL cholesterol. Large buoyant LDL particles increase heart disease risk by 44% and small LDL particles raise heart disease risk by 63% as demonstrated in a 2009 paper by Mora and associates.[22]

Both saturated fat and cholesterol cause oxidative stress which directly feeds cancer cells, as demonstrated by Levy et al.[23]

Compare that with Elkan et al.'s findings that a vegan diet reduces both LDL and oxidized LDL, as shown in their randomized 2008 review, and it is clear that saturated fat has an ugly relationship with LDL cholesterol.[24]

"A gluten-free vegan diet in RA induces changes that are potentially atheroprotective and anti-inflammatory, including decreased LDL and oxLDL levels and raised anti-PC IgM and IgA levels."

In 2009, Tonstad and her team asked the question, "What is the prevalence of type 2 diabetes in people following different types of vegetarian diets compared with that in nonvegetarians?" They examined 22,434 men and 38,469 women. They normalized for social class, level of education, age, gender, sleep cycle, illness, diet, physical activity, ethnicity, and BMI.[25] What they found, in their own words, is,

"The 5-unit BMI difference between vegans and nonvegetarians indicates a substantial potential of vegetarianism to protect against obesity. Increased conformity to vegetarian

diets protected against risk of type 2 diabetes after lifestyle characteristics and BMI were taken into account. Pesco- and semi-vegetarian diets afforded intermediate protection."

This is backed up by findings that saturated fats cause obesity and insulin resistance by increasing the levels of circulating non-esterified fatty acids and killing insulin producing beta-cells.[26]

"Western diets rich in saturated fats cause obesity and insulin resistance, and increase levels of circulating NEFAs [non-esterified ('free') fatty acids]. In addition, they contribute to beta-cell failure in genetically predisposed individuals."

"This cellular stress response may thus be a common molecular pathway for the two main causes of Type 2 diabetes, namely insulin resistance and beta-cell loss."

According to a 2013 paper by Estadella and associates, saturated fat can promote lipotoxicity both directly through inflammatory pathways and indirectly through alterations to bacteria in the gut, and that both of these pathways perpetuate a feedback process which elevates the risk factors for various diseases.[27]

A 2006 study led by Nicholls concluded that saturated fat reduces the anti-inflammatory potential of HDL and impairs arterial endothelial function, and that polyunsaturated fat, such as that found in many plant foods, boost anti-inflammatory activity.[28]

The reason all of this is not common knowledge became abundantly clear in 2016 when a lawsuit alleged that the USDA dietary guidelines were established after heaving lobbying by the American Egg Board.[29]

"According to the committee, a Freedom of Information Act request they filed "revealed a money trail from the American Egg Board to universities where DGAC members were employed and persistent industry pressure to weaken cholesterol limits."

In addition to saturated fats, some animal products contain trans fats. According to the official USDA nutrient database, cheese, milk, yogurt, burgers, chicken fat, turkey meat, bologna, and hot dogs contain about 1 to 5 percent trans fats.[30] In 2003, the National Academies of Science (NAS), concluded that there is no safe intake level of trans fats.[31] According to their study,

"…any incremental increase in trans fatty acid intake increases coronary heart disease risk."

IGF-1

IGF, or insulin growth factor, is a set of polypeptide hormones that stimulate cell proliferation. IGF-3, for instance, proliferates only normal cells, whereas IGF-1 will proliferate both normal and malignant cancer cells, as shown by Allen et al. in 2002.[32] The study outlines IGF-1's connection to breast cancer while demonstrating that vegetarians and vegans have the lowest serum levels of the hormone, ergo the lowest risk factor for cancer, respectively. The study's authors write,

> *"There has been some speculation that cow's milk, which naturally contains bovine IGF-I and is identical to human IGF-I, may increase circulating IGF-I levels and thus may affect cancer risk. Indeed, two dietary intervention studies have found a dairy milk supplement to cause a 10% increase in serum IGF-I levels among adults and children."*

Allen's findings were corroborated by a 2009 paper published in Endocrine Reviews, in which Kleinberg, Wood, Furth, and Lee demonstrated a clear positive correlation between IGF-1 and breast cancer.[33]

That same year, Rowlands et al. connected IGF-1 levels to prostate cancer, effectively showing that both men and women are adversely affected by the circulating hormone.[34]

Naomi Allen, who pioneered the research into IGF-1 as a risk factor for cancer, demonstrated as far back as 2000 that vegan men have very low serum levels of IGF-1 but overall healthy levels of bioavailable androgens, the building blocks for hormones.[35]

When we zoom out and look at the human population as a whole, centenarians, or individuals who live beyond 100, exhibit low levels of IGF-1 as shown in this 2009 review by Salvioli et al.[36]

Methionine

Methionine is an essential amino acid. However, overconsumption of methionine has been linked to cancer growth in a number of studies. The foods highest in methionine are meat, dairy, eggs, and fish.

Tumor cells are unable to proliferate beyond the G2 phase without methionine, a requirement called methionine dependence, which was noticed as early as 1993.[37]

Ruiz et al. demonstrated in 2005 that lower levels of methionine are linked with maximum life span in mammals.[38]

This study was followed up four years later by a closer look at humans, in which McCarty and colleagues found that low-methionine vegan diets prove to be a feasible life extension strategy.[39]

More recently, a thorough look at the biochemistry revealed that reactions between glucose and methionine yielding gaseous sulfur-containing compounds give way to tumor malignancy, suggesting that limiting methionine intake could be a new approach to cancer treatment.[40]

In case you have ever wondered, it is this sulfurous odor that is the primary reason dogs can detect cancer through their heightened sense of smell.[41]

Heme Iron

Iron is found in two forms – heme iron which comes from animal sources and non-heme iron which we get from plant sources.

Iron is an essential nutrient but overconsumption can lead to death. A 2010 study by Sharp supported earlier findings that unfortunately, the body has no mechanism of ridding itself of excess iron so choosing your dietary sources is extremely important.[42]

For this exact reason, iron absorption is regulated by the intestines as shown in a 2005 study by Steele, Frazer, and Anderson.[43]

West and Oates found in their hallmark 2008 study that heme iron has the ability to bypass the body's regulatory mechanism, thereby disposing the body to toxic overload.[44]

In a 2012 study by Ward and associates, the researchers demonstrated that heme iron, the type found only in animal products, causes DNA damage and leads to oxidative stress which directly feeds cancer cells. It has been shown repeatedly to promote esophageal cancer by catalyzing endogenous formation of N-nitroso compounds, which are the potent carcinogens also found in cigarettes.[45]

A meta-analysis of 59 epidemiological studies from 1995-2012 by Fonseca-Nunes et al. corroborated this finding 2 years later that heme iron is a significant risk factor for various forms of cancer because it is a pro-oxidant.[46]

Bao and colleagues reported in their 2012 meta-analysis that heme iron is also a significant risk factor for type 2 diabetes.[47]

According to Yang and associates as published in 2014, there is no safe level of heme iron intake.[48] As little as 1mg/day, or only 5% of the daily requirement of iron, was shown to increase risk for coronary heart disease by 27%. They concluded,

"This meta-analysis suggests that heme iron intake was associated with an increased risk of CHD."

Phthalates

Phthalates are both natural and manmade acids that can be found in fatty animal foods such as milk, butter, and meat. They have been shown to disrupt the endocrine system through antiandrogenic pathways.[49]

A 2006 cross-sectional study of Americans found that phthalates are positively associated with obesity, insulin resistance, and type 2 diabetes.[49]

Four years later, Colacino, Harris, and Schecter conducted a similar national review and found equally alarming trends primarily linked to the consumption of poultry and other types of meat, but, to be fair, also found phthalate metabolites in tomatoes and potatoes.[50]

In a 2009 study conducted by Durmaz et al., it was shown that phthalates cause pubertal gynecomastia, or the enlargement of male breasts in adolescence.[51] Additionally, Swan and associates found that prenatal phthalate exposure impairs testicular function, stunts growth of the penis later in life, and contributes to an overall physical feminization of men.[52] Suddenly, eating meat doesn't seem so manly anymore.

That same year, Swan, along with a different team, published another paper on the matter, demonstrating a behavioral abnormality expressed in boys with higher phthalate exposure, stating that they are less prone to play outdoors, to play physically and aggressively, to take risks, and other male-typical play behavior, suggesting an overall docility and lower levels of testosterone.[53]

This was corroborated by parallel findings in 2010 where Cho et al. found that phthalate exposure adversely affects neurodevelopment in children, while citing earlier findings that it has a positive association with delayed development of the reproductive system, reduced birth weight, allergies, and asthma.[54]

The detrimental effects of phthalate exposure are thoroughly documented,[55] with its toxicity often referred to as the "phthalate body burden"[50] because the body is struggling to develop properly despite environmental and dietary exposure.

Animal Proteins

Animal proteins are often touted as healthier and more bioavailable than their plant alternatives. Is there any truth to this claim?

In 2016, Song et al. conducted the largest and longest-running study ever performed comparing animal and plant sources of protein in the human diet consisting of 131,342 participants running for 26 years and found a positive association between animal proteins and cardiovascular death as well as all-cause mortality and an equal and opposite lower risk of death with plant protein consumption.[56]

In 2003, researchers found that soy protein promotes bone and calcium homeostasis in postmenopausal women, effectively strengthening bones in a section of the population particularly at risk for osteoporosis, whereas milk protein was found responsible for leaching 33% more calcium compared to baseline levels thereby increasing women's risk for bone loss.[57]

When it comes to muscular gains, a 2013 study compared whey and rice protein side by side for performance and strength training and found no distinguishable difference between the two groups, concluding that rice protein was just as effective at building muscle as whey.[58]

In 2015, Babault, et al. found that pea protein actually promoted a greater increase in muscle gains as compared to whey protein and a placebo control.[59]

A causal link between consumption of milk protein and s-insulin and insulin resistance was established in late 2004, characterizing a risk factor for type 2 diabetes.[60]

Heavy Metals

Most people, by now, are aware of the dangers of heavy metal bioaccumulation in seafood, like mercury, lead, and arsenic[61, 62] for instance, so we are not going to cover that here. However, most people are not aware of a similar phenomenon that occurs in the bones of livestock. It is this reason that bone broth, as advocated heavily in the paleo diet community, has alarmingly high levels of lead, as demonstrated by Monro, Leon, and Puri in 2013.[63] It is worth noting that the study used organic chickens.

Various sources of heavy metals in meat comprise an overall elevated risk factor as compared to plant foods. This includes hunters who prefer to shoot and kill their own wild game, as studies have shown that bullet fragments elevate lead exposure to dangerous levels, such as a study from 2009 titled Lead Bullet Fragments in Venison from Rifle-Killed Deer: Potential for Human Dietary Exposure.[64]

Parasites and Miscellaneous Toxins

According to a study published in 2013,[65] the dangers of meat consumption include,

> *"Issues like the presence of various toxic contaminants, including the most commonly found persistent organic pollutants or POPs (dioxins, polychlorinated biphenyls (PCBs); polyaromatic hydrocarbons (PAH) in smoked products, heteroaromatic amines (HAA) in cooked products, and leukotoxin diols in comminuted meat products. A number of other potentially toxic compounds are also possible to identify and quantify in meat and meat products."*

This includes aflatoxins, nitrites and nitrates, choline, carnitine, methylamines, endotoxins, parasites, etc.

Of the 24 common dietary parasites that humans can contract, fully 22 of them are **only** contracted from eating animals (the other two parasites are only contracted through plants or seaweed that has been contaminated from animal sources). However, to be technical, there are 277 known species of tapeworms that are contracted by eating animals, although we only counted them once. One interesting thing to point out is that all parasite cleansing regimens have one thing in common: they are all plant-based remedies.

You might be thinking, "Fine, I'll just cook my meat until all the parasites are killed." Unfortunately, that does not solve anything. In a paper published in 2009, it was shown that consumption of meat causes endotoxemia, an instantaneous inflammatory response caused by dead bacteria that are carried by lipid cells to reach the stomach.[66] These dead bacterial cells are not destroyed by cooking, stomach acid, or pancreatic enzymes.

Additionally, cooking meat creates genotoxic carcinogens, such as PhIP which has been linked to breast cancer and other forms of cancer, as demonstrated by Lauber and Gooderham in 2011.[67]

Bear in mind that a study published in the Lancet in December 2015 concluded that red meat consumption constitutes a possible carcinogen and that processed meat such as hot dogs, ham, sausages, and meat-based sauces cause colorectal cancer, findings endorsed by the World Health Organization.[68]

Dispelling Dietary Dogma

It is paramount that the roots of knowledge grow deep in the minds of the uninformed if we wish to dispel dietary dogma from discussion. You can no longer deny it; Animal products contain a multitude of things that have been empirically shown to adversely affect our health. You may have noticed that of all the risk factors we just explored, none of them mattered whether the animal product in question was organic, free range, growth hormone free, or antibiotic-free. These meaningless distinctions seem to disarm and allure consumers into thinking they are somehow safer.

Choosing not to use animal products not only behooves you, it is vastly more sustainable for the environment as animal agriculture is the primary reason for deforestation, species extinction through habitat destruction, ocean dead zones, water pollution, and excessive water consumption.[69] Moreover, as reported by the Cornell Chronicle in 1997, the United States alone could feed 800 million additional people with the grain that we instead feed to livestock.[70]

The full scope of the environmental and sustainability argument for veganism is so voluminous that it was not included in this book. However, the material is in the public domain for anyone who wishes to explore this aspect further. There is, of course, an equally significant ethical argument for veganism which we will explore in Chapter Seven.

I simply cannot cover every risk factor for animal products in this book alone, but I tried to hit on the major ones here to convey the general idea that animal products are unfit for human consumption. For every study I referenced throughout the book so far, there are easily hundreds more backing up each one.

CHAPTER II
IS DIETARY CHOLESTEROL NECESSARY?

Despite over 40 years of repetitive medical findings demonstrating a clear causal link between dietary cholesterol and heart disease, many people still assert that dietary cholesterol is not only safe, it is in fact healthy.[71]

Whereas established science has weighed in consistently with warnings about the toxicity of cholesterol for nearly half a century, many people insist that the handful of studies that contradict this "consensus" are the honest studies worthy of scholarly attention.

Cholesterol proponents often decry the established science as a conspiracy perpetrated by the statin industry seeking to boost sales in a war against cholesterol. While it is a compelling hypothesis, no one can point to any specific examples to support this claim.

In Chapter One, we demonstrated the toxicity of cholesterol. Now, let us proceed to answer the next most common question, "Is dietary cholesterol necessary?"

Phytosterols versus Dietary Cholesterol

Many cholesterol proponents push multiple claims forward at once, some true, some false, attempting to weave together a seemingly convincing argument.

For instance, a common argument goes like this: cholesterol is needed to perform certain functions in the body, plant foods have their own form of cholesterol and this is evidence that humans can consume cholesterol safely; however, animal products are the best source of cholesterol.

Let's pick this apart one claim at a time and see how well the thesis holds up.

Through a process called cholesterol biosynthesis, your liver will produce all the cholesterol that your body needs. Period. You do not need any from your diet. The less cholesterol you eat, the more your body will produce. This is known as a cholesterol baseline and everyone's is different.

Animal products are technically the only dietary sources of cholesterol. While plants do contain a toxic nutriment called phytosterol which is structurally similar to cholesterol, the human body has evolved mechanisms to block its absorption in the intestines because the body recognizes its toxicity.

Moreover, plant phytosterols have ironically been shown to lower LDL cholesterol absorption in the intestine in many studies, as pointed out by Gylling and Simonen in 2015, effectively lowering the risk of coronary heart disease. [72]

It is this lack of dietary cholesterol and the LDL reduction from plant phytosterols that cause vegans to exhibit lower LDL cholesterol levels than omnivores, as first established by Sanders and Roshanai in 1992.[73]

MYTH: Eskimos Have Extremely High Cholesterol and Enjoy Optimal Health

You may have heard the myth about the healthy Eskimo. Cholesterol proponents often point out that the Inuit peoples living in the Arctic subsist almost exclusively on a carnivorous diet and yet they enjoy abundant health and longevity despite having an average cholesterol score of 200mg/dl compared to the optimal range of 50-70mg/dl, as O'Keefe et al. demonstrated in 2004.[74]

Now, supposing this is true, *and we'll get to the reasons why it's not in a moment*, this still would speak more to some sort of metabolic adaptation specific to the Inuit people and not to humanity as a whole. Different environments have different selective pressures that might cause genetic variance within a species. However, we must rigorously test a hypothesis with available data to see if it holds any water.

Since the Eskimos lived in isolation for roughly 6,000 years until the mid-1800s, cholesterol proponents argue that they had lived healthy lives until they were introduced to western diets. However, we know this is not the case because we have strong evidence that directly contradicts these claims.[75]

In 2013, Thompson et al. published a review of mummified remains of Eskimos dating back 2,000 years that displayed extensive atherosclerosis of the heart, brain, and limbs.[76] Anthropologists found the frozen remains of two women, one that died in her 20s and one that died in her 40s, both from heart disease, displaying premature death in the only examples we have of ancient Eskimo remains.

The life expectancy of Eskimos is 12 to 15 years shorter than Canadians who are some of their nearest neighbors.[77] Moreover, the life expectancy of Canadians climbs each year whereas the life expectancy of Eskimos is stagnant and falls increasingly further behind.[78]

This is in large part due to the anomalously high rates of atherosclerosis, osteoporosis[79], cancer, and parasite infection[80] observed in Eskimo populations. In fact, persistent organic pollutant (POP) body burdens and heavy metal toxicity is such an issue that scientists have found Eskimos exhibit levels 8-10 times higher than non-Eskimos.[81] Inuit women have been found to have levels of PCB's in their breast milk 5- 10 times higher than women in southern Canada.

Cholesterol proponents have conflated the mere survival of the Eskimos with actual thriving.

Smith-Lemli-Opitz Syndrome

Smith-Lemli-Opitz syndrome, or SLOS, is a genetic metabolic disorder that inhibits cholesterol production in the body. SLOS only affects 1 out of every 60,000 babies.[82] However, there is an 80% prenatal or perinatal mortality rate meaning most babies do not even survive. Those that do survive are often left with mental retardation, physical deformities, and other health complications.

The desperation of cholesterol proponents is fairly obvious when they reach for a genetic mutation that affects a small fraction of the population as evidence that dietary cholesterol is necessary for the general population.[82]

This rare syndrome inhibits the body's production of the enzyme DHCR7 which in turn causes a buildup of the sterols 7DHC and 8DHC in serum at thousands of times higher than optimal levels. In fact, cholesterol lowering statin drugs is often how doctors treat SLOS patients because they help to lower 7DHC levels, as discussed by Svoboda et al. in 2012.[83]

While SLOS is often cited for inhibiting cholesterol production, this is not always the case, as Porter demonstrated in 2008 that SLOS patients can exhibit completely normal levels of cholesterol synthesis.[84] Essentially, scientists are unsure of whether or not cholesterol plays any part at all in the symptoms expressed by SLOS patients.[85]

Combined, these findings render this entire argument invalid.

Case Study: Healthy Adult Male Exhibiting Extremely Low Cholesterol

There exist other genetic abnormalities that we can look to in our investigation that are even rarer than SLOS which also cause extremely low cholesterol levels.

Take, for example, this 1979 case study of a man afflicted with asymptomatic familial hypobetalipoproteinemia which caused his LDL cholesterol baseline to be just 4-8mg/dl as well as HDL levels at half the normal levels.[86] He was described as having "remarkably good health" and exhibited no detectable secondary symptoms.

Although individuals genetically disposed to low cholesterol are at no greater risk for illness or disease, there are simple ways for these individuals to raise their cholesterol levels if they want to without relying on animal products. According to the American Heart Association,

"Some tropical oils, such as palm oil, palm kernel oil and coconut oil, also can trigger your liver to make more cholesterol."[87]

CHAPTER III
ANATOMICAL EVIDENCE DEMONSTRATING THAT HUMANS ARE HERBIVORES

In Chapter One, we explored the medical data illustrating the many health risks of consuming animal products. Now, we will evaluate the anatomical evidence supporting the conclusion that human beings are categorically herbivorous animals. The question of our taxonomical classification is really one of evolutionary biology. Fortunately, scientists have identified obvious physical distinctions among mammals that are dead giveaways as to whether a particular animal is naturally designed to eat meat, plants and meat, or just plants.

As Milton R. Mills, M.D. points out in The Comparative Anatomy of Eating,

"Humans are most often described as "omnivores." This classification is based on the "observation" that humans generally eat a wide variety of plant and animal foods. However, culture, custom and training are confounding variables when looking at human dietary practices. Thus, "observation" is not the best technique to use when trying to identify the most "natural" diet for humans. While most humans are clearly "behavioral" omnivores, the question still remains as to whether humans are anatomically suited for a diet that includes animal as well as plant foods.

A better and more objective technique is to look at human anatomy and physiology. Mammals are anatomically and physiologically adapted to procure and consume particular kinds of diets. (It is common practice when examining fossils of extinct mammals to examine anatomical features to deduce the animal's probable diet.)

> *Therefore, we can look at mammalian carnivores, herbivores (plant-eaters) and omnivores to see which anatomical and physiological features are associated with each kind of diet. Then we can look at human anatomy and physiology to see in which group we belong."*[88]

40 Anatomical Features that Classify Humans as Herbivores

There are several types of features that help biologists determine the feeding behaviors of animals.[89] For instance, digestive abilities, "hunting or gathering" abilities, reproductive habits, locomotive abilities, and circadian rhythms are all factors taken into consideration. To illustrate this better, here are two simple examples. Stomach acidity differs greatly between herbivores, omnivores, and carnivores, which would demonstrate an animal's evolutionary adaptation to digest simple carbohydrates such as fruit or complex proteins and fats such as meat. Additionally, whether or not an animal has claws will likely determine if it uses them for hunting or not.

It is important that a conclusion is not reached after reviewing one or two data points. Rather, we must make our conclusion by assessing the totality of all available data. To conclude humans are anything other than herbivores is to ignore the following striking pieces of evidence. The following list includes anatomical features and dietary adaptations.

1) Carnivores have facial muscles that are reduced to allow a wide mouth gap to swallow large chunks of meat or entire animals whole. Omnivores' facial muscles are also reduced. However, herbivores and humans have in common well-developed facial muscles for chewing plant matter.

2) Both carnivores and omnivores have a jaw angle that is acute. Both herbivores and humans have an expanded jaw angle.

3) The location of the jaw joint in carnivores and omnivores is on the same plane as their molar teeth. The location of the jaw joint in herbivores and humans is above the plane of the molars.

4) The jaw in carnivores and omnivores is designed to shear and has minimal side-to-side motion. The jaw in herbivores and humans is very dexterous and moves side-to-side and front-to-back.

5) The major jaw muscle in carnivores and omnivores is the temporalis. The major jaw muscles in herbivores and humans are the masseter and pterygoids.

6) The size comparison between mouth opening and head size is very exaggerated in carnivores and omnivores. However, in herbivores and humans the mouth opening to head size is quite small.

7) In carnivores and omnivores, the incisor teeth are short and pointed. In herbivores and humans, the incisor teeth are broad, flattened, and spade-shaped.

8) In carnivores and omnivores, the canine teeth are long, sharp, and curved. In herbivores, the canine teeth are dull and usually short, although sometimes they are long for defense. Other times, herbivores have no canines at all. In humans, they are short and blunted. It is worth pointing out that just because we refer to our own teeth as canines, does not mean they have anything in common with actual canines in carnivores and this name has more to do with their location on the jaw.

9) In carnivores and omnivores, their molar teeth are sharp, jagged, and blade-shaped. In herbivores, they are flattened with cusps or have a complex surface. In humans, they are flattened with nodular cusps.

10) Carnivores do not chew their food; they swallow it whole. Omnivores swallow food whole or perform simple crushing before swallowing. Herbivores and humans require extensive chewing before swallowing food.

11) The saliva in carnivores and omnivores contains no digestive enzymes whatsoever. The saliva in herbivores and humans contains carbohydrate digesting enzymes.

12) Carnivores and omnivores have what is called a "simple" stomach. Herbivores can either have simple stomachs or stomachs with multiple chambers. In this case, humans have simple stomachs. However, the pH of carnivore and omnivore stomachs is less than or equal to 1. In herbivores and humans, the stomach pH is between 4 and 5.

13) The stomach capacity of carnivores and omnivores is roughly 60% to 70% of the total volume of the digestive tract. In herbivores, it is less than 30% of the total volume of the digest tract. In humans and frugivores, or animals that only eat fruit, it is 21% to 27% the total volume of the digestive tract.

14) Carnivores have a liver that is proportionally 50% larger than others. Omnivores have a liver that is proportionally larger than herbivores.

Herbivores have a liver that is proportionally larger than frugivores. Frugivores and humans have the smallest livers.

15) In carnivores and omnivores, the length of the small intestine is 3 to 6 times the body length, measured from neck to anus. In herbivores, the length of the small intestine can measure 10 to 12 times the body length, and sometimes more. In humans, the small intestines are 10 to 11 times the body length.

16) Carnivores and omnivores have colons that are simple, short, and smooth. Herbivores have colons that are long, complex, and may be sacculated. Humans have colons that are long and sacculated.

17) Carnivores and omnivores can detoxify preformed vitamin A from food with their liver. Herbivores and humans cannot and require pro-vitamin A carotenoids.

18) Carnivores and omnivores have kidneys that produce extremely concentrated urine. Herbivores and humans produce moderately concentrated urine.

19) Carnivores and omnivores have bile flow that is comparatively moderate to heavy. Herbivores and humans have bile flow that is comparatively weak.

20) The kidneys of carnivores and omnivores produce urate oxidase, or uricase. The kidneys of herbivores and humans do not.

21) The colons of carnivores and omnivores are alkaline. The colons of herbivores and humans are acidic.

22) For carnivores and omnivores, peristalsis does not require fiber to stimulate. For herbivores and humans, it does.

23) Carnivores and omnivores can metabolize large amounts of cholesterol efficiently. Herbivores and humans can only metabolize phytosterols efficiently.

24) Carnivores require approximately 2 to 4 hours to digest a meal. Omnivores require approximately 6 to 10 hours to digest a meal. Herbivores require approximately 24 to 48 hours to digest a meal. Frugivores and humans require approximately 12 to 18 hours to digest a meal.

25) Carnivores and omnivores cannot convert short chain fatty acids into long chain fatty acids. Herbivores and humans can.

26) Carnivores and omnivores have sharp claws. Herbivores have flattened nails or blunt hooves. Humans have flattened nails.

27) Carnivores and omnivores have zonary-shaped placentas. Herbivores and humans have discoid-shaped placentas.

28) Carnivores and omnivores cool themselves by panting and only have sweat glands in their paws if they have paws. Herbivores and humans have sweat glands all over their bodies.

29) Carnivores and omnivores are 100% covered in hair. Herbivores and humans have pores with extensive hair covering their bodies.

30) Carnivores and omnivores have multiple teats for nursing litters of offspring. Some herbivores also have multiple teats. Frugivores and humans have dual breasts for nursing one to two offspring.

31) Carnivores, omnivores, and herbivores walk on all fours. Humans and many frugivores walk upright or at least have the ability to do so.

32) Carnivores, omnivores, and some herbivores produce vitamin C endogenously. Frugivores, some herbivores, and humans must consume vitamin C through their diet.

33) Carnivores require taurine in their diet which is found in most animal tissues such as muscle, viscera, and brain but is not found in plants. Humans and most omnivores and herbivores synthesize taurine endogenously.[90]

34) Carnivores and omnivores do not have prehensile arms, hands, feet, or tails. Herbivores and humans do.

35) The brains of carnivores and omnivores are fueled by fats and proteins. The brains of herbivores and humans are fueled by glycogen.

36) Carnivores and omnivores do not have full-color vision. Herbivores and humans have full-color vision.

37) Humans and herbivores sleep approximately 8 hours per 24-hour cycle, whereas carnivores and omnivores spend approximately 18 to 20 hours sleeping per 24-hour cycle.

38) Carnivores and omnivores drink by lapping their tongue. Herbivores and humans drink by sipping with their upper lip.

39) Carnivores are generally adapted for short sprints to catch their prey. Herbivores are generally adapted for endurance to outlast and outrun their predators. Humans are adapted for endurance (with the assistance of the aforementioned sweat glands).

40) Male carnivores do not have seminal vesicles as part of their reproductive anatomy. Male herbivores and male humans do have seminal vesicles. Erectile dysfunction is more often seen in men with elevated cholesterol levels[91] and high levels of LDL "bad" cholesterol.[92]

More anecdotally, our closest primate relatives eat an almost exclusively vegan or frugivorous diet. Also, ironically, the number one cause of choking deaths in humans is from eating meat according to a 2007 study by Dolkas et al.[93]

The Evolution of Binocular Vision

A false assertion made my meat proponents is that humans have binocular vision which proves we are designed to hunt. In 1974, Matt Cartmill proposed the Visual Predation Hypothesis which essentially states that prey species typically have eyes on the sides of their heads to look out for predators, while predators have evolved binocular vision to stalk their prey.[94]

If we examine our pre-hominid ancestors starting with Dryomomys some 55 million years ago, which was essentially a tree-dwelling shrew, which did not have forward facing eyes but was arguably our first ancestral creature to switch from eating insects to eating fruit. Around the same time period, Carpolestes, similar to today's wooly possum, also had eyes that were not forward facing. Nonetheless, it had teeth that were highly specialized for eating flowers, seeds, and fruit.[95]

Then came Notharctus at 45 million years ago, similar to a modern-day lemur, whose diet consisted primarily of fruit and leaves based on the fossil remains we have of its teeth. This was our first primate-like ancestor and it just so happened to have evolved binocular vision – not for hunting, but for navigating tree branches easier in the forest canopy as it leaped long distances high up in the air. This is known as the Arboreal Locomotion Hypothesis.[95]

There are a few exceptions to this hypothesis, such as squirrels which live in trees but have eyes on the sides of their heads. However, some have pointed out that the only exceptions to this rule are smaller mammals, concluding that there is a larger selective pressure for larger animals who stand to risk greater injury if they fall from the treetops.

Some biologists posit that binocular vision was also imperative for early primates to begin manipulating plant foods, such as twisting and plucking fruit from branches or peeling it. According to a 2004 paper by R. A. Barton entitled *Binocularity and brain evolution in primates,*

> *"Fine-grained stereopsis is likely to be critical for the visually guided, delicate manipulation of plant foods, which has been proposed as a key adaptation of ancestral primates."*[96]

Approximately 30 million years ago, Aegyptopithecus emerged, similar to a modern day howler monkey, which had eyes even closer together on the front of its face. Both Aegyptopithecus and the howler monkey are considered herbivores and predominantly eat fruit.[95]

What we see is a complete inversion of Cartmill's Visual Predation Hypothesis. In fact, during the period of time where our early ancestors evolved binocular vision, they actually adapted from a diet consisting mostly of insects to one consisting mostly of fruit. In the same time frame, our ancestors evolved from having claws to having fingernails and they lost their overlapping predatory molars used for shearing flesh and snapping bones (or insect carcasses) and developed in-line molars for grinding plant matter. Additionally, our vision and smell dulled, both of which are highly refined for predators.

In 2008, Changizi and Shimojo published a report called "X-Ray Vision" and the Evolution of Forward Facing Eyes, which is perhaps the most compelling hypothesis to date.[97] In their own words it states,

> *"...the degree of binocular convergence is selected to maximize how much the mammal can see in its environment. Mammals in non-cluttered environments can see the most around them with panoramic, laterally directed eyes. Mammals in cluttered environments, however, can see best when their eyes face forward, for binocularity has the power of "seeing through" clutter out in the world. Evidence across mammals closely fits the predictions of this "X-ray" hypothesis."*

In fact, the scientists actually found a direct correlation between the relative degree of how leafy an animal's environment is and the distance between its eyes. This is especially true for predators in the ocean such as sharks, dolphins, and octopi which have eyes on the sides of their heads but have no problems finding and killing their prey. Moreover, many large herbivorous mammals have eyes on the front of their heads including koalas, tree kangaroos, and sloths.

Diets of Early Hominids and Brain Development

Meat proponents like to attribute humans' rapid brain development with eating meat. Of all the arguments put forward by meat proponents, this one is perhaps the silliest. There are countless species that have consumed meat for much longer than humans and our early hominid ancestors. In fact, many species have eaten an exclusively carnivorous diet for millions of years longer than us. Why aren't sharks, crocodiles, or tigers the smartest species on the planet?

In 2014, Melin and associates published a review in the Journal of Human Evolution claiming that the change of seasons and the quest for elusive bugs spurred tool use and problem-solving skills among primates.[98] Although they may have been on the "hunt" for insects, this likely comprised less than five percent of their overall diet, the rest consisting of fruit, leaves, seeds, and flowers.

Another hypothesis was postulated by Harvard biologist Richard Wrangham that stated the sudden and dramatic availability of calories and carbohydrates through our use of fire to cook food afforded early hominids the ability to more adequately meet their nutritional needs and provide much more fuel for their brains. Fire happens to be a tool unique to humans and has played a major role in our diet for quite some time.

According to Smithsonian Magazine,

"[Wragham's colleague Rachel] Carmody explains that only a fraction of the calories in raw starch and protein are absorbed by the body directly via the small intestine. The remainder passes into the large bowel, where it is broken down by that organ's ravenous population of microbes, which consume the lion's share for themselves. Cooked food, by contrast, is mostly digested by the time it enters the colon; for the same amount of calories ingested, the body gets roughly 30 percent more energy from cooked oat, wheat or potato starch as compared to raw, and as much as 78 percent from the protein in an egg."[99]

A California study published in the Journal of Nutrition in 1999 concluded that,

"Anthropoids, including all great apes, take most of their diet from plants, and there is general consensus that humans come from a strongly herbivorous ancestry. Though gut proportions differ, overall gut anatomy and the pattern of digestive kinetics of extant apes and humans are very similar. Analysis of tropical forest leaves and fruits routinely consumed by wild primates shows that many of these foods are good sources of hexoses, cellulose, hemicellulose, pectic substances, vitamin C, minerals, essential fatty acids, and protein. In general, relative to body weight, the average wild monkey or ape appears to take in far higher levels of many essential nutrients each day than the average American and such nutrients (as well as other substances) are being consumed together in their natural chemical matrix. The recommendation that Americans consume more fresh fruits and vegetables in greater variety appears well supported by data on the diets of free-ranging monkeys and apes."[100]

Atherosclerosis Only Affects Herbivores

In Chapter One, we looked at the causal relationship between dietary cholesterol and coronary heart disease,[101] multiple types of cancer,[102, 103, 104] and Alzheimer's.[105] Now, let's examine the various ways scientists know that cholesterol causes atherosclerosis, a disease that scientists are only able to create in herbivores.

At the 39th Annual Williamsburg Conference on Heart Disease[106] held in 2012, medical doctors Mina Benjamin and William Roberts pointed out that while there are 10 risk factors for atherosclerosis, or narrowing of the arteries, 9 of these factors are contributory at most but do not cause the disease in and of themselves. The only risk factor known to cause atherosclerosis is dietary cholesterol.

After spending 50 years researching coronary heart disease, William Roberts published his four key findings proving that this disease manifests from the consumption of cholesterol.[106]

1. ***"Atherosclerosis is easily produced experimentally in herbivores (monkeys, rabbits) by giving them diets containing large quantities of cholesterol (egg yolks) or saturated fat (animal fat).*** *Indeed, atherosclerosis is one of the easiest diseases to produce experimentally, but the recipient must be an herbivore. It is not possible to produce atherosclerosis in carnivores (tigers, lions, dogs, etc.). In contrast, it is not possible to produce atherosclerosis simply by raising a rabbit's blood pressure or blowing cigarette smoke in its face for an entire lifetime.*

2. ***Atherosclerotic plaques contain cholesterol.***

3.   *Societies with high average cholesterol levels have higher event rates (heart attacks, etc.) than societies with much lower average cholesterol levels.*

4.   *When serum cholesterol levels (especially the low-density lipoprotein cholesterol [LDL-C] level) are lowered (most readily, of course, by statin drugs), atherosclerotic events fall accordingly and the lower the level, the fewer the events* ("less is more"). *Although most humans consider themselves carnivores or at least omnivores, basically we humans have characteristics of herbivores.*"

Individuals who have a cholesterol score between 50mg and 70mg per dl do not develop atherosclerosis[8] whereas a cholesterol score above 75mg/dl causes the progression of atherosclerosis and this relationship is linear, as in the higher the cholesterol score the faster the atherosclerotic progression.[9]

Incidence of Chronic Diseases Unseen in Predominantly Vegetarian Societies

In a 2007 article published in the Baylor University Medical Center Proceedings, William Roberts, M.D. also pointed out the following.

"Some extremely common conditions in the Western world are relatively uncommon in purely or predominantly vegetarian and fruit-eating societies. These include 1) severe atherosclerosis and its devastating consequences (heart attacks, brain attacks, etc.); 2) systemic hypertension: in societies that eat minuscule amounts of salt, the systemic arterial blood pressure is usually about 90/60 mm Hg, a level near what it is at birth but a level in the Western world often associated with shock; 3) stroke; 4) obesity; 5) diabetes mellitus; 6) some common cancers (colon, breast, prostate gland); 7) constipation, cholecystitis, gallstones, appendicitis, diverticulosis, hemorrhoids, inguinal hernia, varicose veins; 8) renal stones; 9) osteoporosis and osteoarthritis; 10) salmonellosis and trichinosis; and 11) cataracts and macular degeneration."[107]

A 2014 meta-analysis conducted by Lap Tai Le and Joan Sabaté published in the Journal of Nutrients reviewed thirteen articles involving hundreds of thousands of participants in total. They concluded,

"In summary, vegetarians have consistently shown to have lower risks for cardiometabolic outcomes and some cancers across all three prospective cohorts of Adventists. Beyond meatless diets, further avoidance of eggs and dairy products may offer a mild additional benefit. Compared to lacto-ovo-vegetarian diets, vegan diets seem to provide some added

protection against obesity, hypertension, type-2 diabetes; and cardiovascular mortality. In general, the protective effects of vegetarian diets are stronger in men than in women."[108]

In 2013, Tantamango-Bartley and colleagues performed an analysis on the prevalence of cancer between vegetarian and non-vegetarian groups to assess animal products as dietary risk factors.[109]

"We examined the association between dietary patterns (non-vegetarians, lacto, pesco, vegan, and semi-vegetarian) and the overall cancer incidence among 69,120 participants of the Adventist Health Study-2. Cancer cases were identified by matching to cancer registries. Cox proportional hazard regression analysis was conducted to estimate hazard ratios, with "attained age" as the time variable."

They concluded that vegetarian diets offer protection against multiple forms of cancer. In their own words,

"When analyzing the association of specific vegetarian dietary patterns, vegan diets showed statistically significant protection for overall cancer incidence in both genders combined and for female-specific cancers."

Red Meat and Mortality

A 28-year study conducted by Pan et al. which ran from 1980 to 2008 examined 121,342 participants to determine the health risk, if any, that red meat consumption poses to humans.[110] In total, they documented 23,926 deaths and 2.96 million person-years of aggregate data. Suffice to say, this study has attained the gold-standard of medical evaluation.

"We prospectively followed 37698 men from the Health Professionals Follow-up Study (1986-2008) and 83644 women from the Nurses' Health Study (1980-2008), who were free of cardiovascular disease (CVD) and cancer at baseline. Diet was assessed by validated food-frequency questionnaires and updated every four years."

The study's authors concluded that red meat consumption is associated with an increased risk of cardiovascular disease mortality, cancer mortality, and all cause mortality. Additionally, they found that substitution of other healthy protein sources for red meat is associated with a lower mortality risk.

The exact numbers that the team estimated for the risk factors were quite alarming. At just one serving increase per day of unprocessed red meat, total lifetime mortality rose by 113%. For cardiovascular disease mortality, one serving increase of red meat raised the hazard ratio by 118% for men and 121% for women. For cancer, the hazard ratio was raised by 110% for men and 116% for women.

Substituting for just one serving of red meat per day with fish, poultry, nuts, legumes, low-fat dairy, or whole grains resulted in a 7% to 19% reduction in mortality risk. The authors also estimated that 9.3% of male deaths and 7.6% of female deaths could have been prevented if all individuals consumed less than half a serving per day of red meat.

If the first three chapters of this book have convinced you to try out a plant-based diet, but you are worried that it won't meet your body's nutritional needs, in Chapter Four we will investigate whether or not this fear is supported by the scientific community.

CHAPTER IV
ARE VEGANS AT A HIGHER RISK FOR NUTRITIONAL DEFICIENCIES?

So you're considering giving up animal products in favor of a plant based diet, but you keep running into self-proclaimed experts who want to scare you that vegans are at a higher risk for nutritional deficiencies. You know, like Vitamin A, B_{12}, iron, D_3, EPA, DHA, K_2, and invariably, protein. But what does the science say? Do vegans have any reason to be concerned? Okay, let's take these one at a time.

Vitamin A

Vitamin A is a fat-soluble vitamin that is found preformed in animal products or is synthesized in your body from pro-vitamin A carotenoids, like beta carotene.[111]

While it is true that Vitamin A from animal sources are used more readily by the body, as shown in a 2010 study by Tang, absorption rate is virtually a non-issue for vegans because pro-vitamin A carotenoids are found in such great abundance in a balanced plant-based diet.[112] Vegans typically reach their bodies' Vitamin A demands within one or two meals.

A 2006 study by Penniston and Tanumihardjo found that toxicity levels of preformed Vitamin A can be reached at just twice the daily recommended intake, whereas your liver will regulate the production of Vitamin A when you consume pro-vitamin A carotenoids and toxicity is "largely impossible."[113] In other words, it is easy to overdose on vitamin A from animal products but impossible to do so from plant sources.

It is worth noting that there exists an inverse correlation between BMI and the beta carotene conversion factor.[112] In other words, the more body fat an individual has, the lower their capability to convert beta carotene into vitamin A. A vegan of normal BMI will synthesize vitamin A without any issues.[114]

Vitamin B12

Vitamin B12, the largest and most complex vitamin,[115] is a water soluble vitamin produced by algae found in fresh water[116] and is also found in healthy soil.[117]

While it is wise for vegans to eat fortified foods or to consume B12 supplements,[118] meat eaters are also consuming B12 supplements indirectly because livestock feed is supplemented with B12 to keep animals healthy.[119] This is not exclusively a vegan deficiency, nor is it exclusively a human deficiency. It does, however, speak to a soil crisis with much larger implications for modern industrial farming.

Eating animals does not naturally meet your body's B12 needs – this only occurs when farmers introduce it artificially into livestock feed. So why don't we, the humans, just take the supplements directly and avoid the cholesterol and saturated fats that are found in meat? Now that's food for thought.

Iron

To recap what we covered in Chapter One, iron is found in two forms – heme iron which comes from animal sources and non-heme iron which we get from plant sources.

Iron is an essential nutrient but too much can lead to death. A 2010 study by Sharp supported earlier findings that unfortunately, the body has no mechanism of ridding itself of excess iron so choosing your dietary sources is extremely important.[42]

For this exact reason, iron absorption is regulated by the intestines as shown in a 2005 study by Steele, Frazer, and Anderson.[43]

West and Oates found in their hallmark 2008 study that heme iron has the ability to bypass the body's regulatory mechanism, thereby disposing the body to toxic overload.[44]

In a 2012 study by Ward and associates, the researchers demonstrated that heme iron, the type found only in animal products, causes DNA damage and leads to oxidative stress which directly feeds cancer cells.[45] It has been shown repeatedly to promote esophageal cancer by catalyzing endogenous formation of N-nitroso compounds, which are the potent carcinogens also found in cigarettes.

A meta-analysis of 59 epidemiological studies from 1995-2012 by Fonseca-Nunes et al. corroborated this finding 2 years later that heme iron is a significant risk factor for various forms of cancer because it is a prooxidant.[46]

Bao and colleagues reported in their 2012 meta-analysis that heme iron is also a significant risk factor for type 2 diabetes.[47]

According to Yang and associates as published in 2014, there is no safe level of heme iron intake. As little as 1mg/day, or only 5% of the daily requirement of iron, was shown to increase risk for coronary heart disease by 27%.[48] They concluded,

> *"This meta-analysis suggests that heme iron intake was associated with an increased risk of CHD."*

So, if iron from animal products has no safe limit, the next logical question is: do people who follow plant-based diets get a sufficient amount of non-heme iron? Saunders, et al. concluded in 2013 that they "are not at any greater risk of iron deficiency."[120]

Vitamin D3

Vitamin D3 is a fat-soluble hormone produced in the skin when it receives UVB sunlight.[121]

Generally speaking, 90% is produced by the body and 10% is consumed through diet, so if an individual is deficient in vitamin D, it makes much more sense to address this by spending more time outdoors than through one's diet.

As of 2011, 41.6% of Americans were found to be deficient in vitamin D[122] although only 2.5% of Americans were vegan that same year,[123] thereby reaffirming that this is not a dietary problem, it is a lifestyle problem.

According to the National Institutes of Health, as little as 5-30 minutes of midday sun exposure per week is enough to prevent symptoms of deficiency.[121]

Additionally, there are a number of bioavailable plant sources for vitamin D such as sun-exposed mushrooms or lichen.

When you combine this with the fact that dairy products are fortified with vitamin D, just like we discussed with B12, it makes more sense to supplement directly than to consume animal products that are artificially fortified.

It is worth noting that the darker your skin and the higher BMI you have, the more sunlight you need to produce adequate levels of D3.[124]

EPA & DHA

EPA, or eicosapentaenoic acid, and DHA, or docosahexaenoic acid, are both omega-3 fatty acids that are important for the brain, heart, joints, and eyes, among other things,[125] although a 2009 study by Sanders found that "there is no evidence of adverse effects on health or cognitive function with lower DHA intake in vegetarians."[126]

While there are both plant-based and animal-based dietary sources of preformed EPA and DHA, our body has a mechanism to convert alpha linolenic acid, a shorter omega-3 found in plant oils, into EPA and DHA.

Because microalgae are one of the most prolific sources of dietary EPA and DHA, it is widely believed that fish are the best source of these nutrients for humans, therefore vegans are deficient.

A 2008 paper by Welch, et al. found that the conversion of ALA into EPA and DHA was actually 22% greater in vegetarians than in fish-eaters, demonstrating how the body will create more of these omega-3 fatty acids if need be.[127]

Still, meat proponents will claim that because the ALA conversion to DHA is only 3.8%, this is somehow not enough for vegans to meet their needs, which is simply untrue.[128] As little as one tablespoon of flax oil or 3oz of walnuts, for instance, would be enough to meet the daily recommended intake, without taking into account the rest of the food consumed that day.

A 2012 study by Oken, et al. reminds us that while fish contain essential fatty acids, they are rich sources of methylmercury and other toxicants and are inferior sources of EPA and DHA compared to plants.[129]

Not only that, but Bao et al. found in 2013 that consumption of nuts were associated with decreased risk of cancer, heart disease, respiratory disease, and all-cause mortality.[130]

Rizos and colleagues published a meta-analysis in 2012 demonstrating that fish oil supplementation was not associated with a lower risk of all-cause mortality and heart disease.[131]

Vitamin K2

Vitamin K2 is a fat soluble vitamin that is produced endogenously in the body and can also be acquired through diet. It plays a role in bone strength and heart health.[132]

Certain vegan foods are actually the best sources of K2, such as sauerkraut or natto. Natto actually has the highest concentration of K2 of any food we know of. That being said, vitamin K2 is produced by healthy bacteria inside the GI, therefore deficiencies in adults are very rare.[133]

K2 can also be synthesized in arterial walls, the pancreas, and testes. It stays in the bloodstream for long periods of time, which is yet another reason that vegans are unlikely to develop deficiencies.

To put it simply, just like vitamin A, EPA, DHA, collagen, and biotin, your body will produce the vitamin K2 it needs.

It is worth noting that while vitamin K2 improves arterial function,[134] animal products that are high in K2 – such as eggs, milk, cheese, beef, and chicken – are also high in saturated fats which inhibit endothelial cell function[135, 136, 137] and cause coronary heart disease. So eating these animal products negates any benefit of the K2 one would hope to gain from them. This could explain the conflicting research on the benefits of dietary K2.

Although paleo and meat proponents really emphasize the need to supplement K2, only one study, published in the Netherlands in 2004, has been put forward showing that K2 supplementation could possibly reduce the risk of heart disease and the findings were admittedly weak.[138] However, a German study by Nimptsch, et al. found the exact opposite – that K2 supplementation actually posed a greater risk for heart disease.[139]

Protein

First of all, let's refute the misconception that animal proteins are better for you than plant proteins. In 2016, Song et al. conducted the largest study ever performed comparing animal and plant sources of protein in the human diet – consisting of 131,342 participants running for 26 years – and found a positive association between animal proteins and cardiovascular death as well as all-cause mortality and lower risk of death with plant proteins.[56]

Okay, next, let's dispel the myth that vegans cannot get enough protein in their normal diet.

The Academy of Nutrition and Dietetics' official stance is,

> *"Vegan diets typically meet or exceed recommended protein intakes, when caloric intakes are adequate."*[140]

Let's also remember that all proteins are originally synthesized by plants. All whole plant foods contain protein and all animals get their protein directly from plants or indirectly by eating other animals.

Allen and associates found in 2002 that plant proteins are better than animal proteins at regulating serum IGF-1 levels which are a risk factor for cancer.[141]

When it comes to muscular gains, a 2013 study compared whey and rice protein side by side for performance and strength training and found no distinguishable difference between the two groups, concluding that rice protein was just as effective at building muscle as whey.[142] Combine this with the fact that plant foods have a complete amino acid profile, as demonstrated by McDougall in 2002, and there is no reason to ever consume animal proteins.[143]

Official Position of the Academy of Nutrition and Dietetics on Plant-Based Diets

According to the Academy of Nutrition and Dietetics,

> *"Well-designed vegetarian diets provide adequate nutrient intakes for all stages of the lifecycle and can also be useful in the therapeutic management of some chronic diseases. Overall nutrition, as assessed by the Alternative Healthy Eating Index, is typically better on vegetarian and vegan diets compared with omnivorous diets.*

Compared to nonvegetarian diets, vegetarian diets can provide protection against many chronic diseases, such as heart disease, hypertension, type 2 diabetes, obesity, and some cancers. Furthermore, a vegetarian diet could make more conservative use of natural resources and cause less environmental degradation."[140]

In 1984, the Oxford study looked at 11,140 participants and found that vegans have a lower risk of heart disease, cancer, diabetes, and all-cause mortality even after adjusting for smoking, BMI, and social class.[144]

Medical Mythology

So, let's recap. Wherever there are nutrients found in animal products, there are better versions of those same nutrients found in vegan products. Contrary to what the myth mongers would have you believe, there are no nutritional deficiencies that exclusively affect vegans.

Sticking to a balanced plant-based diet is not only feasible; it is vastly superior in regard to health, sustainability, and cost. Tofu and other meat alternatives often cost 10 cents on the dollar compared to real meat. Therefore, you are spending more money and going out of your way to poison yourself.

Perhaps a question we might want to ask is why is none of the research cited in this book being promulgated through mainstream outlets? Why is there still the prevailing narrative that we need animal products to stay healthy? Why are the masses still superstitious with the medical mythology that was exposed long ago?

CHAPTER V
MISCONCEPTIONS ABOUT SOY AS A SUBSTITUTE FOR MEAT

One of the most common ingredients used in the substitution of animal products is soy. Some of the soy products that are on the market include soy milk, tofu, tempeh, miso, and soy sauce. There are many myths surrounding this ubiquitous plant food, such as it being one of the leading causes of the feminization of men, it is unsafe for women with breast cancer, or it is an inferior source of protein. Let us now examine the peer-reviewed medical literature and address the actual causes of the feminization of men.

Soy Does Not Adversely Affect Testosterone Levels in Men

What does the scientific community conclude about excessive consumption of soy protein lowering testosterone in men? Thankfully, the medical literature is quite clear on this. A 2010 meta-analysis by Hamilton-Reeves et al. published in the American Society for Reproductive Medicine's journal Fertility and Sterility set out, in their own words,

> *"To determine whether isoflavones exert estrogen-like effects in men by lowering bioavailable T through evaluation of the effects of soy protein or isoflavone intake on T, sex hormone–binding globulin (SHBG), free T, and free androgen index (FAI) in men."*[145]

The study was set up as follows.

"Fifteen placebo-controlled treatment groups with baseline and ending measures were analyzed. In addition, 32 reports involving 36 treatment groups were assessed in simpler models to ascertain the results."

Finally, the team spelled out their conclusion in plain English.

"The results of this meta-analysis suggest that neither soy foods nor isoflavone supplements alter measures of bioavailable T concentrations in men."

Also in 2010, Mark Messina published a meta-analysis concluding,

"The intervention data indicate that isoflavones do not exert feminizing effects on men at intake levels equal to and even considerably higher than are typical for Asian males."[146]

According to a peer-reviewed paper published in 2007 by Kalman et al., soy protein was shown to have no effect on the reproductive hormones of men.[147] Soy was demonstrated to promote lean body mass in men, which also seems to contradict many people's misconception about soy being a poor protein for anabolic muscle production. This was further corroborated 3 years later by two separate studies.[145, 146]

It is worth pointing out that men have far less estrogen receptors than women and that men naturally produce estrogen in the testes, so even if men consume trace amounts of phytoestrogens as is the case with soy, this has little impact on hormonal homeostasis, as demonstrated by Dickson and Clarke in 1981.[148]

To date, very few isolated studies found a disruption in male testosterone but these studies had the participants consuming over 16 servings of soy per day and it is entirely possible that genetic abnormalities played a role in these anomalous results.

Soy Provides Protective Benefits Against Cancer

Soy boasts a number of protective benefits against chronic disease. According to a 2006 study, consumption of soy decreases prostate cancer risk in men and breast cancer risk in women.[149]

*"Suggestive evidence that **soy-rich diets decrease prostate cancer risk**, accords well with the observation that ERbeta appears to play an antiproliferative role in healthy prostate. In the breast, ERalpha promotes epithelial proliferation, whereas ERbeta has a*

*restraining influence in this regard – consistent with the emerging view that **soy isoflavones do not increase breast cancer risk, and possibly may diminish it.***"

Additionally, they found that soy is negatively associated with blood clot-related disorders such as pulmonary embolisms or strokes.

"Hepatocytes do not express ERbeta; this explains why soy isoflavones, unlike oral estrogen, neither modify serum lipids nor provoke the prothrombotic effects associated with increased risk for thromboembolic disorders."

MYTH: Soy Lowers Sperm Count

Another misconception about soy that has contributed to the "soy-boy" stereotype is that it lowers sperm count. This is categorically false and demonstrates how individuals can misinterpret data. The truth is that soy increases seminal fluid production resulting in lower sperm concentration but not lower sperm count. The overall sperm count remains the same. This is backed up by findings from Chavarro, Toth, Sadio, and Hauser in 2008. According to their study,

"Soy food and soy isoflavone intake were unrelated to sperm motility, sperm morphology or ejaculate volume. These data suggest that higher intake of soy foods and soy isoflavones is associated with lower sperm concentration."[150]

Soy Consumption is Safe for Infants and Children, Bovine Milk is Not

A 2014 study conducted by Vandenplas and associates reported that when administering soy-based infant formulas, which were introduced over 100 years ago, they "did not find strong evidence of a negative effect on reproductive and endocrine functions." Additionally, the researchers said, "Wherever possible, a meta-analysis was carried out." Finally, they added,

"The patterns of growth, bone health and metabolic, reproductive, endocrine, immune and neurological functions are similar to those observed in children fed CMF (cow's milk formula) or HM (human milk)."[151]

This study mirrored identical results 13 years prior in 2001 by Strom et al. The stated objective of the study was "To examine the association between infant exposure to soy formula and health in young adulthood, with an emphasis on reproductive health." They concluded,

"Exposure to soy formula does not appear to lead to different general health or reproductive outcomes than exposure to cow milk formula. Although the few positive findings should be explored in future studies, our findings are reassuring about the safety of infant soy formula."[152]

So what about infant exposure to cow's milk? In 1999, Vaarala and colleagues demonstrated,

"Cow's milk feeding is an environmental trigger of immunity to insulin in infancy that may explain the epidemiological link between the risk of type 1 diabetes and early exposure to cow's milk formulas."[153, 154]

In a paper published in the New England Journal of Medicine in 1992, researchers found that cow's milk triggers an autoimmune response that attacks the pancreas.[155] They demonstrated that early exposure to bovine milk destroys insulin-producing beta cells produced in the pancreas which contributes to the development of diabetes. The researchers concluded,

"This likens the disease in humans to that in diabetes-prone rodents, in which the prevention of exposure to cow's milk early in life prevents the development of the disease."

Soy Consumption Safe for Women

According to Chen et al.'s 2014 meta-analysis, soy consumption is safe for women including pre- and post-menopausal women and those battling breast cancer.[156] This overturns the common misconception that certain women should avoid soy at all costs. Their conclusion was,

"We meta-analyzed more and newer research results, and separated women according to menopausal status to explore soy isoflavone-breast cancer association. We founded that soy isoflavone intake could lower the risk of breast cancer for both pre- and post-menopausal women in Asian countries. However, for women in Western countries, pre- or post-menopausal, there is no evidence to suggest an association between intake of soy isoflavone and breast cancer."

In 2003, researchers found that soy protein promotes bone and calcium homeostasis in postmenopausal women, effectively strengthening bones in a section of the population particularly at risk for osteoporosis, whereas milk protein was found responsible for leaching 33% more calcium compared to baseline levels thereby increasing women's risk for bone loss.[157]

True Causal Factors in the Feminization of Men

Now that we have looked at what the medical literature has to say about soy, we will address how the paranoia around soy is a red herring for the truly feminizing dietary and environmental risk factors that men should be aware of. These risk factors include consumption of poultry and beer, exposure to phthalates such as BPA and BPS, and lifestyle problems such as inadequate sleep, use of anabolic steroids, consumption of highly fatty foods, and obesity.

Contrary to popular belief, testosterone levels in males do not naturally decline after age 40. Kelsey et al. proved this when they published a peer-reviewed paper in 2014 entitled *A Validated Age-Related Normative Model for Male Total Testosterone Shows Increasing Variance but No Decline after Age 40 Years.*[158] In healthy males, testosterone peaks around age 19, drops until approximately age 40, and then plateaus thereafter. The vast amount of men who continue to see T levels drop after age 40 are likely being exposed to dietary and environmental factors that play a role in blocking testosterone production. They concluded,

> *"We show that total testosterone peaks [mean (2.5–97.5 percentile)] at 15.4 (7.2–31.1) nmol/L at an average age of 19 years, and falls in the average case [mean (2.5–97.5 percentile)] to 13.0 (6.6–25.3) nmol/L by age 40 years, but we find no evidence for a further fall in mean total testosterone with increasing age through to old age."*

As we discussed in Chapter One, phthalates are both natural and manmade acids that can be found in fatty animal foods such as milk, butter, and meat. Poultry is the highest dietary source of phthalates. They have been shown to disrupt the endocrine system through antiandrogenic pathways and are often referred to as "gender-bender chemicals."[49]

A 2006 cross-sectional study of Americans found that phthalates are positively associated with obesity, insulin resistance, and type 2 diabetes. There, you have a secondary risk factor as obesity has been linked repeatedly to lower testosterone levels, such as in this 2014 study by Fui, Dupuis, and Grossman entitled *Lowered testosterone in male obesity: mechanisms, morbidity and management.*[159] Moreover, high-fat meals have been shown to reduce testosterone concentrations without affecting luteinizing hormone.[160]

Soy opponents often point out that testosterone has dropped dramatically in the west in the last 20 years, while the domestic soy industry has swelled from $200 million annually to $3 billion. However, correlation does not equal causation and this superficial evaluation ignores the fact that obesity has skyrocketed from 10% in 1960 to over 34% by 2012, according to the CDC.[161]

In 2010, Colacino, Harris, and Schecter conducted a national review and found that poultry and other types of meat contain the highest concentrations of phthalates but, to be fair, also found phthalate metabolites in tomatoes and potatoes. However, phthalate metabolites are not as potent as phthalates.[50]

In a 2009 study conducted by Durmaz et al., it was shown that phthalates cause pubertal gynecomastia, or the enlargement of male breasts in adolescence.[51] Additionally, Swan and associates found that prenatal phthalate exposure impairs testicular function, stunts growth of the penis later in life, and contributes to an overall physical feminization of men.[52] Suddenly, eating meat doesn't seem so manly anymore.

Finally, we can look to a 2009 study in which Maruyama, Oshima, and Ohyama traced consumption of bovine milk to decreased testosterone as a result of the exogenous estrogen inherent in cow's milk.[162]

For more, please refer to the phthalates section of Chapter One.

Alcohol Consumption Lowers Testosterone

Beer contains hops which have isoflavones that behave more detrimentally in the body than those in soy. Hops contain a phytoestrogen named 8-PN which is thousands of times more potent than those found in soy, as pointed out by Possemiers et al. in the Journal of Agriculture and Food Chemistry in 2005.[163]

This is partly due to the fact that 8-PN bonds with alpha receptors as pointed out by Schaefer et al. in 2003[164] whereas soy bonds with beta receptors as demonstrated by McCarty in 2006.[149] It is this very reason that soy could potentially help prevent gynecomastia, or the development of "man boobs," because when the isoflavones in soy bond with beta receptors in breast tissue it turns off cell proliferation. This is the same pathway by which soy prevents breast cancer. According to the study,

> *"In the breast, ERalpha promotes epithelial proliferation, whereas ERbeta has a restraining influence in this regard — consistent with the emerging view that soy isoflavones do not increase breast cancer risk, and possibly may diminish it."*

Compare this with the aforementioned findings by Durmaz et al. in 2009 that demonstrated phthalates, such as those found in poultry, cause pubertal gynecomastia, or the enlargement of male breasts in adolescence.[51] Poultry consumption causes "man boobs" whereas soy prevents against it.

In 1979, Ellingboe and Varanelli found that ethanol inhibits testicular testosterone production.[165] This means any distilled alcohol fermented from grain, fruit, or vegetables lowers testosterone levels. This also includes many popular soft drinks and fruit drinks as well as various processed foods.[166]

That same year, Van Thiel and colleagues discovered that alcohol causes testicular atrophy in rodents, although this does not necessarily correlate in humans as rodent models are not directly indicative of human results.[167] Van Thiel also confirmed liver cirrhosis as a pathogenic mechanism for the feminization of men in human trials.[168]

As early as 1983 in the journal Alcoholism: Clinical and Experimental Research, the doctors pointed out that,

> *"Male gonadal dysfunction produced by liver cirrhosis has been recognized for decades. The association of testicular atrophy, gynecomastia, and liver cirrhosis was described initially by Corda and Silvestrini."*[169]

This journal has dozens of studies linking alcohol consumption to lower testosterone for those wishing to explore further.[170]

CHAPTER VI
REASONS TO AVOID HONEY

Of all the animal products that vegans abstain from in their diet, honey is arguably the least understood and often the most trivialized by non-vegans. Even some self-professed "vegans" consume honey, royal jelly, and propolis, regardless of the fact that these are not vegan foods. Insects belong to the animal kingdom so anything insects produce is without question an animal byproduct. Regardless, most consumers only hear about the health benefits of consuming honey and not the health risks. Moreover, most people are simply unaware of the amount of honey bees that are killed in the beekeeping industry.

Toxic Compounds Found in Honey

Let's begin with the lesser known health risks of honey consumption. In 2013, Islam and associates published a paper in the Journal of Applied Toxicology entitled *Toxic Compounds in Honey*.[171] In this thorough analysis, the researchers broke with the orthodox reporting of honey's health benefits and dared to ask the question, "Are there any health risks associated with honey consumption?" They found a number of risk factors, both natural and artificial, that should give consumers pause the next time they are in the sweetener aisle. The researchers summarized their findings as such,

> *"There is a wealth of information about the nutritional and medicinal properties of honey. However, honey may contain compounds that may lead to toxicity. A compound not naturally present in honey, named 5-hydroxymethylfurfural (HMF), may be formed during the heating or preservation processes of honey. HMF has gained much interest, as*

it is commonly detected in honey samples, especially samples that have been stored for a long time. HMF is a compound that may be mutagenic, carcinogenic and cytotoxic. It has also been reported that honey can be contaminated with heavy metals such as lead, arsenic, mercury and cadmium. Honey produced from the nectar of Rhododendron ponticum contains alkaloids that can be poisonous to humans, while honey collected from Andromeda flowers contains gray anotoxins, which can cause paralysis of limbs in humans and eventually leads to death. In addition, Melicope ternata and Coriaria arborea from New Zealand produce toxic honey that can be fatal. There are reports that honey is not safe to be consumed when it is collected from Datura plants (from Mexico and Hungary),belladonna flowers and Hyoscamus niger plants (from Hungary), Serjanialethalis (from Brazil),Gelsemium sempervirens (from the American Southwest), Kalmia latifolia, Tripetalia paniculata and Ledum palustre. Although the symptoms of poisoning due to honey consumption may differ depending on the source of toxins, most common symptoms generally include dizziness, nausea, vomiting, convulsions, headache, palpitations or even death. It has been suggested that honey should not be considered a completely safe food."

Moreover, the chemical composition of honey is not exactly a nutritious food, to put it mildly. Bee products contain sugar, animal proteins, and fat. Although there are some healthy sugars, humans lack the enzymes to break down the acids that give honey its shelf-stable qualities.

In an article entitled *Why Honey is a Harmful Food* authored by Dr. T. C. Fry,

"As a food for us, honey is woefully mineral and vitamin deficient. Humans require infinitely more food factors than bees. While honey contains several very desirable sugars, these have been rendered toxic by the protective acids imparted to them by the bees. These acids are the bees' preservatives. Humans do not have the enzymes to break these acids down, as have the bees, and must rob their bodies of vital base-forming minerals to neutralize the acids.

When humans eat honey, it immediately begins to reabsorb moisture from the stomach and stomach flora. It destroys our symbiotic bacterial population wholesale. Several tablespoons of honey makes most people very sick.

In humans, honey, more so than cane and beet sugars, is acid-forming and decalcifying. The body draws calcium from its teeth and bones, if necessary, to neutralize the acids introduced and formed. Manite acid of honey is a protoplasmic poison. It interacts with protein and from this, forms alcohol, ammonia and carbonic acid.

As eaten, honey is an atrocious food. It is usually added to starches and proteins as a sweetener. It readily ferments when held up in the stomach with other longer-digesting

foods. The byproducts alcohol, ammonia, and carbonic acid are deleterious to human health."[172]

The above risk factors constitute a small overview of some of the medical reasons one might avoid honey to one degree or another. Without going into great detail, this chapter is intended to provide a broad overview of the reasons many vegans avoid honey.

Externalities of Industrial Beekeeping

Most consumers seem to be under the impression that beekeeping is harmless to bees, that the human beekeepers and bees work symbiotically with each other, and that it is of great benefit to the environment given that bees are pollinators.

Bees will not make honey unless a queen is present. Through a cruel process of slowly squishing male bees until semen bursts out for extraction, they will artificially inseminate the mail-order queen bees to begin the process of honey production. Upon arrival, beekeepers rip the wings off of the queen bee to prevent her from flying away. Many queen bees are injured or killed in the transportation process, as are the worker bees anytime a hive is relocated. Some beekeepers within the industry kill off their hives entirely before winter.

There is a common misconception that honeybees are the best pollinators in North America. Honeybees are not actually native to North America. They are in fact an invasive species that were introduced by humans. Many other pollinator species have been severely diminished in numbers by diseases that honeybees brought with them.[173, 174] Additionally, honeybees are territorial and ward off other species from pollinating in the same areas, including "keystone" species.[175]

Finally, commercial pollination and commercial honey production are two disparate industries. According to Justin Schmidt and Stephen Buchmann, Research Entomologists at the USDA Carl Hayden Bee Research Center, the bees that produce the honey are not the same bees that perform the pollination.

"Beekeepers may brag about the importance of honeybees in the necessary transfer of pollen, but many are not involved in the practical aspects of the service… Bees cannot be expected to feed themselves, much less produce any surplus honey while engaged in commercial pollination."[176]

Independent studies have concluded that honeybees are only responsible for pollinating approximately 15% of all crops,[177, 178] whereas the USDA estimates they are responsible for closer to 80%. Since this is a large margin of error, the jury is out on the exact role that honeybees play in the pollination of our environment.

Ethical Considerations

In Chapter Seven, we will explore the ethical argument for veganism, but there are a few ethical points worth mentioning about honey consumption while we are on the subject. Ethics are universal, consistent standards that we can apply to everyone equally. If ethics are not universal, then they are simply a form of tyranny. To remain consistent with the principles of nonviolence and non-exploitation, vegans must include honey in their list of foods to abstain from. Otherwise, what is the point of professing a principle if one allows exceptions? This would seem to give way to a slippery slope.

For whatever reason, many people seem to become focused on defining the boundaries of veganism. Bees, oysters, jellyfish, and other animals are often debated as to whether or not they are fair game. Intelligence, the ability to feel pain, and other considerations are usually proposed as traits to include or exclude certain animals. We will cover this extensively in Chapter Seven.

Regardless, countless studies have confirmed the extraordinary intelligence of bees. For example, bees use a "waggle dance" to convey the location and proximity of wildflowers using vector calculus and physics.[179] It has been documented that bees will adjust their dance every four minutes to account for the one degree change in the angle of the sun.

As consumers, we often become detached from the essence of our food sources, or we never learn exactly what it is that we are eating and why. This holds true with bee products, as many people are unaware of how bees make honey. Honey is produced when bees swallow nectar, regurgitate it, chew it and mix it with their saliva, and swallow it again. This process repeats itself approximately fifty times before the bee vomits the honey as food for their offspring, food for the adults to endure winter, and it is used for hive insulation.

Perhaps animal rights activist Gary Yurofsky said it best.

> *"We lie to ourselves. We play euphemism games. The standard diet of a meat, dairy, and egg eater is blood, flesh, veins, muscles, tendons, cow secretions, things that come out of a hen's ass, and bee vomit."*

CHAPTER VII
A PHILOSOPHICAL PROOF FOR THE ETHICAL SUPERIORITY OF VEGANISM

Until now, we have covered the medical argument for veganism, building upon over 100 peer-reviewed scientific papers. Now, we will address the ethical argument for veganism using syllogistic reasoning. This chapter will not appeal to your emotions outright, because our emotions generally follow our decisions about the morality of the topic at hand. Since we must first establish the morality of the exploitation of animals, we will begin by logically proving why veganism is more ethical than needlessly causing the suffering and death of animals.

From the start, it is important to point out that whether or not you believe, ontologically speaking, morality is intrinsic or whether it is derived from a social contract, we will make the case that to have an internally consistent system for human morality, one cannot exclude animals.

The Minimization of Unnecessary Harm Caused to Animals

Veganism is defined as the minimization of unnecessary harm caused to animals. I want to define this term clearly up front because vegans are often held to a perfect standard and criticized if there is an unavoidable amount of harm that they cause such as the death of insects in agriculture. Since perfection is an impossible standard, veganism is about striving to minimize this harm as much as reasonably possible.

Veganism is about the non-aggression principle which states that any initiation of force is unethical. Self-defense is justified because it is a response to someone else initiating force on you. Therefore, if you are being attacked by a dog, you are justified in fighting back. If the integrity of your house is being compromised by termites and your safety is on the line, you are justified in fighting back. These actions are permissible within the ethics of veganism.

Lesser Value Does Not Justify Violence or Exploitation

To formulate a philosophically consistent system of practical ethics that justifies the slaughter, impregnation, enslavement, and exploitation of animals, one must demonstrate a very clear distinction why these acts are immoral to also carry out on other humans.

From this point forward, when we say "killing" we will imply the unnecessary initiation of force because we are not talking about killing out of self-defense or survival, which are the only justifiable reasons for killing.

To argue that killing humans is immoral whereas killing animals is simultaneously amoral, one must name the trait that excludes animals from this universal principle of the right to life.

Put differently, if you hold the position that humans should not be killed because they have moral value, then you must prove that animals do not also have moral value so as to justify killing them.

Carnists, or individuals who support animal slaughter and exploitation, often misinterpret this with the idea that humans are equal in value with animals. Let us dispel this notion quickly because it is a straw man. Most vegans do not actually think that animals are of equal value to humans; however, this value disparity does not justify slaughter.

I can value my life more than I value yours, but that does not justify me killing you. It is not contradictory to believe that animals are of lesser value and that we should still protect their well-being.

To give a different example, my BMW may be more valuable than my neighbor's Toyota, but that value disparity does not justify me vandalizing his car.

Name the Trait

When you ask a carnist to name the distinguishing trait that justifies the killing of animals and not humans, a number of faulty examples are named. To be clear, this is a logical consistency test and not a proof for compassion, per se. Let's examine the common traits carnists put forward one at a time and discover why each one is false by virtue of a double standard.

If you are to argue that **intelligence** is the trait, then to be consistent you must exclude mentally handicapped humans from the right to life.

If you are to argue that **capacity for language** is the trait, then to be consistent you must exclude humans who are mute from the right to life. This example would also have to ignore the fact that many animals do have language skills.

If you are to argue that **consciousness** is the trait, then to be consistent you must exclude comatose patients from the right to life.

If you are to argue that **bipedalism** is the trait, then to be consistent you must exclude amputees from the right to life. This example would also have to ignore the fact that there are other creatures, such as the kangaroo, that are in fact bipedal.

This logical algorithm goes on to rule out the following traits: *culture/tradition, civilization, ownership, in-group preference, self-conception, future-conception, convenience, uncertainty, tastiness, nutrition, emotionality, capacity to feel pain, religion, science, philosophy, bred to die, circle of life, feeling grounded, capacity to reciprocate morality,* and *value,* as we already discussed.

Appeal to Nature Fallacy

Although the science is extremely clear that human beings are anatomically herbivorous, let's say you reject that data and believe that humans are omnivores. Still, this does not justify eating animals. The ethical dilemma arises due to the fact that humans can live long, healthy lives on a plant-based diet according to the official position of the Academy of Nutrition and Dietetics.[140] In other words, humans eat meat for enjoyment, not for basic survival.

To draw a moral imperative from anatomy is an *appeal to nature* fallacy, which takes the following structure:

- *Humans CAN eat animals, therefore humans SHOULD eat animals.*

This sidesteps around the subject of ethics, which is at the heart of our thesis. Moreover, this argument could also be used to justify cannibalism, because without the aforementioned trait, humans are indistinguishable from animals.

If you accept this *appeal to nature* as part of your argument, then the following statement would be ethically correct:

- *Humans CAN wage war, therefore humans SHOULD wage war.*

Animals Lack Moral Agency

The *appeal to nature* fallacy also encompasses the concept of moral agency. Often, carnists will argue that because a lion kills its prey, it is moral for humans to kill their prey, too. In this assertion, a non-moral agent (the lion) is being compared to a moral agent (the human) without a hint of irony.

The glaring problem is that we do not hold humans who lack moral agency accountable for crimes, such as toddlers or individuals who are certifiably crazy. This is because toddlers and the mentally insane do not understand the consequences of their actions, and neither do animals. Therefore, this argument does not stand to reason.

Also, by this same logic, anything else that lions do is justifiable for humans to do, also. The argument looks like this:

- *Lions do X, therefore humans do X.*
- *Lions kill one another in competition for mates, therefore humans can kill each other in competition for mates.*

Appeal to History Fallacy

Sometimes, carnists assert that a certain benefit was historically derived from animal consumption, such as the misconception that meat consumption was responsible for human brain growth,[99] (*although many researchers believe it was our use of tools in the quest of hard to reach insects that spurred advanced neurodevelopment*).[180] From the assumption that meat was responsible for our neurodevelopment, they then attempt to derive a moral principle from this supposed historical benefit.

The argument goes like this:

- *Humans used to X which may have helped us evolve, therefore X is moral.*
- *Humans used to enslave other humans which may have helped the economy, therefore enslaving other humans is moral.*

Evolution does not determine ethical principles. Tribal warfare has been an intrinsic factor in the natural selection of our species for much longer than meat consumption has been a part of our diet, but this does not morally justify warfare per se.

The Flaw with Subjective Morality

If a carnist rejects morality altogether or claims that morality is subjective, then at the very least they are being consistent. However, they are now rejecting their own right to life, and their own preferences can be trampled on anytime another person's preferences clash with their own. Moreover, moral relativists cannot prove that they are the morally superior ones either, vis-à-vis the lack of an empirical moral standard.

This train of thought is common among post-modernists and nihilists. If someone really wants to make the case for moral relativism, then they must abdicate the ability to criticize veganism since truth and morality are subjective. Therefore, it follows that if you accept an objective system of morality, you can rely on absolute principles to protect your right to life and the right to life of animals.

All too often, cognitive dissonance causes meat eaters to become offended when they are encouraged by vegans to live compassionately. Carnists generally retaliate with a tu quoque fallacy, condemning the vegan for taking the moral high ground. If morality is subjective, how can a carnist logically condemn a vegan for anything?

One example of a subjective moral argument goes like this:

- *Killing and exploiting animals is not wrong if the animals were treated well.*
- *Raping another human is not wrong if the human was treated well.*

Animals Experience Emotions, Pain, and Some Critical Thought

It's self-evident to say that animals are not voluntarily consenting to their own murder, enslavement, imprisonment, impregnation, etc. This is demonstrated by their resistance, their cries for help, their fear, postpartum sadness, and so on. There have also been studies that have measured the intelligence,[181] emotions,[182] and empathy[181] of various animals and found that they are remarkably impressive in all three capacities.

Often, Orwellian doublespeak is used to describe killing an animal, referring to it as "humane slaughter." This oxymoron is not only self-contradictory, it exposes the underlying methods and motivations of carnists who seek to justify the heinous act of slaughter through anthropomorphization.

On the one hand, the word "humane" implies that we should treat animals as humans. On the other hand, we should slaughter them.

Is it also humane to put the fear of death into a creature in the moments before they die? Is it also humane for them to witness their family members being slaughtered?

Aside from the obvious contradiction of choosing certain animals to love and protect as pets while discriminating against other species, this idea of humane slaughter is akin to consensual rape or peaceful war. It is not internally consistent.

The Plant Sentience Argument

Often, meat-eaters will put forward the argument that plants also have consciousness and vegans cannot claim to be more moral because there is no superiority or inferiority to be ascribed to different types of organisms. They use scientific findings such as the Baxter Effect to prove that plants are also sentient beings. For argument's sake, let's go with that and assume that plants are conscious, too.

Veganism already proves more ethical because infinitely fewer plants are killed if you are eating them directly and are not raising livestock. We need not go any further. Also, many types of vegetables are not killed when they are harvested. Rather, a portion of the plant is harvested. This includes foods like broccoli, kale, and cauliflower.

If you really want to take the stance that plants are sentient, too, then fruit proves to be the most ethical food source because fruit is voluntarily offered by the plant to be consumed for the very purpose of spreading its seeds. *It is a symbiotic relationship.* The reason plants put so much time, effort, vitamins, minerals, resources, and energy into the production of a fruit is not so that it will fall and rot, but so that animals will be lured into eating it so that they can help the plant proliferate since the plant cannot move on its own.

This is the evolutionary purpose of fruit bearing. Again, the plant would not allocate all of its resources and effort to fruit-bearing for it to go to waste. Nature is not wasteful; it is efficient and optimal. You could say that we are invited by the plant to enjoy what it offers, but not as a free gift. Instead, it is a mutual transaction, or an equal exchange.

If you are still unconvinced that plants want you to consume their fruit (or flowers, seeds, etc.) then I recommend looking into interspecific competition and the Gause Principle. One particular example is when plants compete to offer the best smelling, brightest, most vibrant and most colorful flowers to attract pollinators.

If we ascribe consciousness to plants, then veganism is morally superior to animal consumption. Extending the practice of compassion to animals is more ethical than intentionally causing them harm.

The inescapable conclusion after rigorous philosophical scrutiny is that if all else is held equal, vegans are more ethical than individuals who consciously consume animal byproducts or otherwise support the exploitation of animals – the same way that if you can prove human-on-human murder is wrong, then if all else is held equal, non-murderers are more ethical than murderers.

CHAPTER VIII
TYING IT ALL TOGETHER

Throughout this book, we asked the question "Are animal products healthy to eat?" The short answer is no, but even with the hundreds of studies cited throughout this book, I have barely scratched the surface of the published medical literature that overwhelmingly supports this conclusion.

In writing this book, it was my hope to teach a couple of secondary lessons outside the scope of nutrition. There are multiple parties deliberately funding junk science[5] or just honestly misconstruing data. Not a lot of people read scientific literature, which is fine – I'm not saying everyone needs to – but those of us that don't have our work cut out for us.

I caution everyone to exercise discernment when listening to dietary and medical advice, even with my research. Taking accountability for your health is the first step in reclaiming the direction of your life, but do so with the understanding that there is an industry built upon the exploitation of your ignorance on these matters.

For those that contribute to and financially support the animal holocaust, your actions are not only unsustainable, they are unethical. Now that you have heard the medical and ethical arguments for veganism, the impetus is on you to change. Perhaps this is the first time you have encountered this information. For those who have never been exposed to the truth before, a moral pass can be granted because they were acting on ignorance. However, anyone who decides not to change their behavior after learning the truth is axiomatically unethical.

Consuming animal products needlessly causes the suffering and death of animals. Now that you have seen the science and ethical dilemma, the impetus is on you to change. Whatever your reason for consuming animal products, be it tradition, taste, or an irrational fear of inadequate nourishment, you no longer have any excuse. You're not tough because you eat meat, and it's not cool to be flippant about causing suffering and death.

For a variety of sadistic reasons, many individuals gleefully make a mockery of the compassion that vegans strive to act on. Individuals who think it is feminine to demonstrate compassion are themselves maladjusted to a depraved culture. For those that attempt to justify eating meat because it makes you feel "grounded," a shocking amount of cognitive dissonance is required for you to feel balanced and connected to the Earth while you consume the slaughtered carcasses of gentle, innocent, and defenseless beings.

The same degree of cognitive dissonance is required when meat eaters feign offense when they are encouraged to live compassionately. Instead they retaliate with a tu quoque fallacy, condemning the vegan for taking the moral high ground and then attempt to criticize the vegan for minor imperfections. Meat eaters who dig their heels in and resist the logic and deny the science of veganism are themselves committed more to convenience than truth and they should be called out for it.

Whether your reason for going plant-based is medical, anatomical, environmental, ethical, or even economical, it is time to make the change.

Perhaps the greatest improvement any one person can make to their diet and health would be to cut out all animal products immediately. Perhaps the greatest impact most of us can have on the environment, the economy, and on world hunger is by going vegan. And perhaps the greatest shift we can make as a species is one towards compassion.

ACKNOWLEDGEMENTS

My mother passed away days before my 26th birthday from a bilateral pulmonary embolism induced by deep leg thrombosis. This means a blood clot formed in her leg which traveled to an artery in her lungs where it obstructed blood flow. A combination of preventable dietary and lifestyle factors contributed to her untimely passing. That event inspired this book. May her untimely passing be not in vain, and serve to save the life of another.

REFERENCES

1.   Jacobs, D. R., Anderson, J. T., & Blackburn, H. (1979). Diet and serum cholesterol: Do ZERO correlations NEGATE the relationship? *American Journal of Epidemiology, 110*(1), 77-87.

2.   de Souza Russell J, Mente Andrew, Maroleanu Adriana, Cozma Adrian I, Ha Vanessa, Kishibe Teruko et al. Intake of saturated and trans unsaturated fatty acids and risk of all cause mortality, cardiovascular disease, and type 2 diabetes: systematic review and meta-analysis of observational studies *BMJ* 2015; 351 :h3978

3.   Jacobs DR Jr, Anderson JT, Blackburn H. Diet and serum cholesterol: do zero correlations negate the relationship? *Am J Epidemiol.* 1979 Jul;110(1):77-87. PubMed PMID: 313701.

4.   Siri-Tarino, P. W., Sun, Q., Hu, F. B., & Krauss, R. M. (2010). Meta-analysis of prospective cohort studies evaluating the association of saturated fat with cardiovascular disease. *The American Journal of Clinical Nutrition, 91*(3), 535–546. http://doi.org/10.3945/ajcn.2009.27725

5.   McDougall, Dr. John. "Ronald M. Krauss, MD—The Doctor Who Made Lard-eating Fashionable." *Dr. McDougall.* March 2014. Web.

6.   Hopkins PN. Effects of dietary cholesterol on serum cholesterol: a meta-analysis and review. *Am J Clin Nutr.* 1992 Jun;55(6):1060-70. PubMed PMID: 1534437.

7.   Clarke, R., Frost, C., Collins, R., Appleby, P., & Peto, R. (1997). Dietary lipids and blood cholesterol: quantitative meta-analysis of metabolic ward studies. *BMJ : British Medical Journal, 314*(7074), 112–117.

8.   James H O'Keefe, Loren Cordain, William H Harris, Richard M Moe, Robert Vogel. Optimal low-density lipoprotein is 50 to 70 mg/dl: Lower is better and physiologically normal, *Journal of the American College of Cardiology,* Volume 43, Issue 11,2004, Pages 2142-2146, ISSN 0735-1097, https://doi.org/10.1016/j.jacc.2004.03.046.

9.   von Birgelen C, Hartmann M, Mintz GS, Baumgart D, Schmermund A, Erbel R. Relation between progression and regression of atherosclerotic left main coronary artery disease and serum cholesterol levels as assessed with serial long-term (> or =12 months) follow-up intravascular ultrasound.

Circulation. 2003 Dec 2;108(22):2757-62. Epub 2003 Nov 17. PubMed PMID: 14623804.

10. Sacks FM, Donner A, Castelli WP, et al. Effect of Ingestion of Meat on Plasma Cholesterol of Vegetarians. *JAMA.* 1981;246(6):640–644. doi:10.1001/jama.1981.03320060042020

11. Gersh, B.J.. (2007). Sequence Variations in PCSK9, Low LDL, and Protection against Coronary Heart Disease. *Yearbook of Cardiology.* 2007. 247-248. 10.1016/S0145-4145(08)70160-6.

12. Brian A. Ference, Wonsuk Yoo, Issa Alesh, Nitin Mahajan, Karolina K. Mirowska, Abhishek Mewada, Joel Kahn, Luis Afonso, Kim Allan Williams, John M. Flack, Effect of Long-Term Exposure to Lower Low-Density Lipoprotein Cholesterol Beginning Early in Life on the Risk of Coronary Heart Disease: A Mendelian Randomization Analysis, *Journal of the American College of Cardiology*, Volume 60, Issue 25, 2012, Pages 2631-2639, ISSN 0735-1097, https://doi.org/10.1016/j.jacc.2012.09.017.

13. Sachdeva A, Cannon CP, Deedwania PC, Labresh KA, Smith SC Jr, Dai D, Hernandez A, Fonarow GC. Lipid levels in patients hospitalized with coronary artery disease: an analysis of 136,905 hospitalizations in Get With The Guidelines. *Am Heart J.* 2009 Jan;157(1):111-117.e2. doi: 10.1016/j.ahj.2008.08.010. Epub 2008 Oct 22. PubMed PMID: 19081406.

14. Kitahara CM, Berrington de González A, Freedman ND, Huxley R, Mok Y, Jee SH, Samet JM. Total cholesterol and cancer risk in a large prospective study in Korea. *J Clin Oncol*. 2011 Apr 20;29(12):1592-8. doi: 10.1200/JCO.2010.31.5200. Epub 2011 Mar 21. PubMed PMID: 21422422; PubMed Central PMCID: PMC3082977.

15. Danilo C, Frank PG. Cholesterol and breast cancer development. *Curr Opin Pharmacol*. 2012 Dec;12(6):677-82. doi: 10.1016/j.coph.2012.07.009. Epub 2012 Aug 3. Review. PubMed PMID: 22867847.

16. Li, Y. C., Park, M. J., Ye, S.-K., Kim, C.-W., & Kim, Y.-N. (2006). Elevated Levels of Cholesterol-Rich Lipid Rafts in Cancer Cells Are Correlated with Apoptosis Sensitivity Induced by Cholesterol-Depleting Agents. *The American Journal of Pathology*, 168(4), 1107–1118. http://doi.org/10.2353/ajpath.2006.050959

17. de la Torre JC. Alzheimer disease as a vascular disorder: nosological evidence. *Stroke*. 2002 Apr;33(4):1152-62. Review. PubMed PMID: 11935076.

18. Esselstyn CB Jr. Resolving the Coronary Artery Disease Epidemic Through Plant-Based Nutrition. *Prev Cardiol*. 2001 Autumn;4(4):171-177. PubMed PMID: 11832674.

19. Esselstyn, C. B. (2007). We Can Prevent and Even Reverse Coronary Artery Heart Disease. *Medscape General Medicine*, 9(3), 46.

20. Elkan, A.-C., Sjöberg, B., Kolsrud, B., Ringertz, B., Hafström, I., & Frostegård, J. (2008). Gluten-free vegan diet induces decreased LDL and oxidized LDL levels and raised atheroprotective natural antibodies against phosphorylcholine in patients with rheumatoid arthritis: a randomized study. *Arthritis Research & Therapy*, *10*(2), R34. http://doi.org/10.1186/ar2388

21. Esselstyn CB Jr, Gendy G, Doyle J, Golubic M, Roizen MF. A way to reverse CAD? *J Fam Pract*. 2014 Jul;63(7):356-364b. PubMed PMID: 25198208.

22. Mora S, Otvos JD, Rifai N, Rosenson RS, Buring JE, Ridker PM. Lipoprotein particle profiles by nuclear magnetic resonance compared with standard lipids and apolipoproteins in predicting incident cardiovascular disease in women. *Circulation*. 2009 Feb 24;119(7):931-9. doi: 10.1161/CIRCULATIONAHA.108.816181. Epub 2009 Feb 9. PubMed PMID: 19204302; PubMed Central PMCID: PMC2663974.

23. Levy Y, Maor I, Presser D, Aviram M. Consumption of eggs with meals increases the susceptibility of human plasma and low-density lipoprotein to lipid peroxidation. *Ann Nutr Metab*. 1996;40(5):243-51. PubMed PMID: 9001684.

24. Elkan AC, Sjöberg B, Kolsrud B, Ringertz B, Hafström I, Frostegård J. Gluten-free vegan diet induces decreased LDL and oxidized LDL levels and

raised atheroprotective natural antibodies against phosphorylcholine in patients with rheumatoid arthritis: a randomized study. *Arthritis Res Ther.* 2008;10(2):R34. doi: 10.1186/ar2388. Epub 2008 Mar 18. PubMed PMID: 18348715; PubMed Central PMCID: PMC2453753.

25. Tonstad, S., Butler, T., Yan, R., & Fraser, G. E. (2009). Type of Vegetarian Diet, Body Weight, and Prevalence of Type 2 Diabetes. *Diabetes Care, 32*(5), 791–796. http://doi.org/10.2337/dc08-1886

26. Cnop M. Fatty acids and glucolipotoxicity in the pathogenesis of Type 2 diabetes. *Biochem Soc Trans.* 2008 Jun;36(Pt 3):348-52. doi: 10.1042/BST0360348. Review. PubMed PMID: 18481955.

27. Débora Estadella, Claudia M. da Penha Oller do Nascimento, Lila M. Oyama, Eliane B. Ribeiro, Ana R. Dâmaso, and Aline de Piano, "Lipotoxicity: Effects of Dietary Saturated and Transfatty Acids," *Mediators of Inflammation*, vol. 2013, Article ID 137579, 13 pages, 2013. doi:10.1155/2013/137579

28. Nicholls SJ, Lundman P, Harmer JA, Cutri B, Griffiths KA, Rye KA, Barter PJ, Celermajer DS. Consumption of saturated fat impairs the anti-inflammatory properties of high-density lipoproteins and endothelial function. *J Am Coll Cardiol.* 2006 Aug 15;48(4):715-20. Epub 2006 Jul 24. PubMed PMID: 16904539.

29.   Lewis, Tanya. "A lawsuit claims government guidelines on cholesterol were tainted by the egg industry." *Business Insider.* January 7, 2016. Web.

30.   Exler, Jacob et al. "Fat and Fatty Acid Content of Selected Foods Containing Trans-Fatty Acids ARS." *USDA Nutrient Data Laboratory.* 1993. Web.

31.   National Academies Press (U.S.). (2003). *Dietary reference intakes for energy, carbohydrate, fiber, fat, fatty acids, cholesterol, protein, and amino acids (macronutrients).* Washington, D.C.: National Academies Press.

32.   Allen NE, Appleby PN, Davey GK, Kaaks R, Rinaldi S, Key TJ. The associations of diet with serum insulin-like growth factor I and its main binding proteins in 292 women meat-eaters, vegetarians, and vegans. *Cancer Epidemiol Biomarkers Prev.* 2002 Nov;11(11):1441-8. PubMed PMID: 12433724.

33.   Kleinberg DL, Wood TL, Furth PA, Lee AV. Growth hormone and insulin-like growth factor-I in the transition from normal mammary development to preneoplastic mammary lesions. *Endocr Rev.* 2009 Feb;30(1):51-74. doi: 10.1210/er.2008-0022. Epub 2008 Dec 15. Review. Erratum in: Endocr Rev. 2012 Dec;33(6):1038. PubMed PMID: 19075184; PubMed Central PMCID: PMC5393153.

34.   Rowlands, M. , Gunnell, D. , Harris, R. , Vatten, L. J., Holly, J. M. and Martin, R. M. (2009), Circulating insulin-like growth factor peptides and

prostate cancer risk: A systematic review and meta-analysis. *Int. J. Cancer*, 124: 2416-2429. doi:10.1002/ijc.24202

35. Allen NE, Appleby PN, Davey GK, Key TJ. Hormones and diet: low insulin-like growth factor-I but normal bioavailable androgens in vegan men. *Br J Cancer*. 2000 Jul;83(1):95-7. PubMed PMID: 10883675; PubMed Central PMCID: PMC2374537.

36. Salvioli, S., Capri, M., Bucci, L. et al. *Cancer Immunol Immunother* (2009) 58: 1909. https://doi.org/10.1007/s00262-008-0639-6

37. Guo HY, Herrera H, Groce A, Hoffman RM. Expression of the biochemical defect of methionine dependence in fresh patient tumors in primary histoculture. *Cancer Res*. 1993 Jun 1;53(11):2479-83. PubMed PMID: 8495409.

38. Ruiz MC, Ayala V, Portero-Otín M, Requena JR, Barja G, Pamplona R. Protein methionine content and MDA-lysine adducts are inversely related to maximum life span in the heart of mammals. *Mech Ageing Dev*. 2005 Oct;126(10):1106-14. PubMed PMID: 15955547.

39. McCarty MF, Barroso-Aranda J, Contreras F. The low-methionine content of vegan diets may make methionine restriction feasible as a life extension strategy. *Med Hypotheses*. 2009 Feb;72(2):125-8. doi: 10.1016/j.mehy.2008.07.044. Epub 2008 Sep 11. PubMed PMID: 18789600.

40. Yamagishi K, Onuma K, Chiba Y, et al. Generation of gaseous sulfur-containing compounds in tumour tissue and suppression of gas diffusion as an antitumour treatment. *Gut* 2012;61:554-561.

41. Pickel, Duane & P. Manucy, Glenda & B. Walker, Dianne & B. Hall, Sandra & C. Walker, James. (2004). Evidence of canine olfactory detection of melanoma. *Applied Animal Behaviour Science* - APPL ANIM BEHAV SCI. 89. 107-116. 10.1016/j.applanim.2004.04.008.

42. Sharp PA. Intestinal iron absorption: regulation by dietary & systemic factors. *Int J Vitam Nutr Res*. 2010 Oct;80(4-5):231-42. doi: 10.1024/0300-9831/a000029. Review. PubMed PMID: 21462105.

43. Steele, T. M., Frazer, D. M. and Anderson, G. J. (2005), Systemic Regulation of Intestinal Iron Absorption. *IUBMB Life*, 57: 499-503. doi:10.1080/15216540500149904

44. West, A. R., & Oates, P. S. (2008). Mechanisms of heme iron absorption: Current questions and controversies. *World Journal of Gastroenterology* : WJG, 14(26), 4101–4110. http://doi.org/10.3748/wjg.14.4101

45. Ward, M. H., Cross, A. J., Abnet, C. C., Sinha, R., Markin, R. S., & Weisenburger, D. D. (2012). Heme iron from meat and risk of adenocarcinoma of the esophagus and stomach. *European Journal of Cancer Prevention*, 21(2), 134–138. http://doi.org/10.1097/CEJ.0b013e32834c9b6c

46. Fonseca-Nunes A, Jakszyn P, Agudo A. Iron and cancer risk--a systematic review and meta-analysis of the epidemiological evidence. *Cancer Epidemiol Biomarkers Prev.* 2014 Jan;23(1):12-31. doi: 10.1158/1055-9965.EPI-13-0733. Epub 2013 Nov 15. Review. PubMed PMID: 24243555.

47. Bao, W., Rong, Y., Rong, S., & Liu, L. (2012). Dietary iron intake, body iron stores, and the risk of type 2 diabetes: a systematic review and meta-analysis. *BMC Medicine*, 10, 119. http://doi.org/10.1186/1741-7015-10-119

48. Yang W, Li B, Dong X, Zhang XQ, Zeng Y, Zhou JL, Tang YH, Xu JJ. Is heme iron intake associated with risk of coronary heart disease? A meta-analysis of prospective studies. *Eur J Nutr.* 2014;53(2):395-400. doi:10.1007/s00394-013-0535-5. Epub 2013 May 26. PubMed PMID: 23708150.

49. Stahlhut RW, van Wijngaarden E, Dye TD, Cook S, Swan SH. Concentrations of urinary phthalate metabolites are associated with increased waist circumference and insulin resistance in adult U.S. males. Environ Health Perspect. 2007 Jun;115(6):876-82. Epub 2007 Mar 14. Erratum in: *Environ Health Perspect.* 2007 Sep;115(9):A443. PubMed PMID: 17589594; PubMed Central PMCID: PMC1892109.

50. Colacino JA, Harris TR, Schecter A. Dietary intake is associated with phthalate body burden in a nationally representative sample. *Environ Health Perspect.* 2010 Jul;118(7):998-1003. doi: 10.1289/ehp.0901712. Epub 2010

Apr 14. PubMed PMID: 20392686; PubMed Central PMCID: PMC2920922.

51.   Durmaz E, Ozmert EN, Erkekoglu P, Giray B, Derman O, Hincal F, Yurdakök K. Plasma phthalate levels in pubertal gynecomastia. *Pediatrics*. 2010 Jan;125(1):e122-9. doi: 10.1542/peds.2009-0724. Epub 2009 Dec 14. PubMed PMID: 20008419.

52.   Swan, S. H., Main, K. M., Liu, F., Stewart, S. L., Kruse, R. L., Calafat, A. M., … the Study for Future Families Research Team. (2005). Decrease in Anogenital Distance among Male Infants with Prenatal Phthalate Exposure. *Environmental Health Perspectives*, 113(8), 1056–1061. http://doi.org/10.1289/ehp.8100

53.   Swan, S. H., Liu, F., Hines, M., Kruse, R. L., Wang, C., Redmon, J. B., … Weiss, B. (2010). Prenatal phthalate exposure and reduced masculine play in boys. *International Journal of Andrology*, 33(2), 259–269. http://doi.org/10.1111/j.1365-2605.2009.01019.x

54.   Cho SC, Bhang SY, Hong YC, Shin MS, Kim BN, Kim JW, Yoo HJ, Cho IH, Kim HW. Relationship between environmental phthalate exposure and the intelligence of school-age children. *Environ Health Perspect*. 2010 Jul;118(7):1027-32. doi:10.1289/ehp.0901376. Epub 2010 Mar 1. PubMed PMID: 20194078; PubMed Central PMCID: PMC2920903.

55. Meeker, J. D., Calafat, A. M. and Hauser, R. (2009), Urinary Metabolites of Di(2-ethylhexyl) Phthalate Are Associated With Decreased Steroid Hormone Levels in Adult Men. *Journal of Andrology*, 30: 287-297. doi:10.2164/jandrol.108.006403

56. Song M, Fung TT, Hu FB, et al. Association of Animal and Plant Protein Intake With All-Cause and Cause-Specific Mortality. *JAMA Intern Med.* 2016;176(10):1453–1463. doi:10.1001/jamainternmed.2016.4182

57. Arjmandi BH, Khalil DA, Smith BJ, Lucas EA, Juma S, Payton ME, Wild RA. Soy protein has a greater effect on bone in postmenopausal women not on hormone replacement therapy, as evidenced by reducing bone resorption and urinary calcium excretion. *J Clin Endocrinol Metab.* 2003 Mar;88(3):1048-54. PubMed PMID: 12629084.

58. Joy JM, Lowery RP, Wilson JM, Purpura M, De Souza EO, Wilson SM, Kalman DS, Dudeck JE, Jäger R. The effects of 8 weeks of whey or rice protein supplementation on body composition and exercise performance. *Nutr J.* 2013 Jun 20;12:86. doi: 10.1186/1475-2891-12-86. PubMed PMID: 23782948; PubMed Central PMCID: PMC3698202.

59. Babault N, Païzis C, Deley G, Guérin-Deremaux L, Saniez MH, Lefranc-Millot C, Allaert FA. Pea proteins oral supplementation promotes muscle thickness gains during resistance training: a double-blind, randomized, Placebo-controlled clinical trial vs. Whey protein. *J Int Soc Sports Nutr.* 2015

Jan 21;12(1):3. doi: 10.1186/s12970-014-0064-5. eCollection 2015. PubMed

PMID: 25628520; PubMed Central PMCID: PMC4307635.

60.   Hoppe C, Mølgaard C, Vaag A, Barkholt V, Michaelsen KF. High intakes

of milk, but not meat, increase s-insulin and insulin resistance in 8-year-old

boys. *Eur J Clin Nutr.* 2005 Mar;59(3):393-8. PubMed PMID: 15578035.

61.   Oken E, Choi AL, Karagas MR, Mariën K, Rheinberger CM, Schoeny R,

Sunderland E, Korrick S. Which fish should I eat? Perspectives influencing

fish consumption choices. *Environ Health Perspect.* 2012 Jun;120(6):790-8.

doi: 10.1289/ehp.1104500. Epub 2012 Feb 22. Review. PubMed PMID:

22534056; PubMed Central PMCID: PMC3385441.

62.   Perelló G, Martí-Cid R, Llobet JM, Domingo JL. Effects of various cooking

processes on the concentrations of arsenic, cadmium, mercury, and lead in

foods. *J Agric Food Chem.* 2008 Dec 10;56(23):11262-9. doi:

10.1021/jf802411q. PubMed PMID: 18986150.

63.   Monro JA, Leon R, Puri BK. The risk of lead contamination in bone broth

diets. *Med Hypotheses.* 2013 Apr;80(4):389-90. doi:

10.1016/j.mehy.2012.12.026. Epub 2013 Jan 31. PubMed PMID: 23375414.

64.   Hunt, W. G., Watson, R. T., Oaks, J. L., Parish, C. N., Burnham, K. K.,

Tucker, R. L., ... Hart, G. (2009). Lead Bullet Fragments in Venison from

Rifle-Killed Deer: Potential for Human Dietary Exposure. *PLoS ONE*, 4(4),

e5330. http://doi.org/10.1371/journal.pone.0005330

65. Püssa T. Toxicological issues associated with production and processing of meat. *Meat Sci.* 2013 Dec;95(4):844-53. doi: 10.1016/j.meatsci.2013.04.032. Epub 2013 Apr 22. Review. PubMed PMID: 23660174.

66. Ghanim H, Abuaysheh S, Sia CL, Korzeniewski K, Chaudhuri A, Fernandez-Real JM, Dandona P. Increase in plasma endotoxin concentrations and the expression of Toll-like receptors and suppressor of cytokine signaling-3 in mononuclear cells after a high-fat, high-carbohydrate meal: implications for insulin resistance. *Diabetes Care.* 2009 Dec;32(12):2281-7. doi: 10.2337/dc09-0979. Epub 2009 Sep 15. PubMed PMID: 19755625; PubMed Central PMCID: PMC2782991.

67. Lauber SN, Gooderham NJ. The cooked meat-derived mammary carcinogen 2-amino-1-methyl-6-phenylimidazo[4,5-b]pyridine promotes invasive behaviour of breast cancer cells. *Toxicology.* 2011 Jan 11;279(1-3):139-45. doi: 10.1016/j.tox.2010.10.004. Epub 2010 Oct 15. PubMed PMID: 20951759.

68. Bouvard V, Loomis D, Guyton KZ, Grosse Y, Ghissassi FE, Benbrahim-Tallaa L, Guha N, Mattock H, Straif K; International Agency for Research on Cancer Monograph Working Group. Carcinogenicity of consumption of red and processed meat. *Lancet Oncol.* 2015 Dec;16(16):1599-600. doi: 10.1016/S1470-2045(15)00444-1. Epub 2015 Oct 29. PubMed PMID: 26514947.

69.   Anderson K, Kuhn K. "The Facts." *Cowspiracy*. Web.

70.   "U.S. could feed 800 million people with grain that livestock eat, Cornell ecologist advises animal scientists." Cornell Chronicle. August 7, 1997. Web.

71.   Jacobs, D. R., Anderson, J. T., & Blackburn, H. (1979). Diet and serum cholesterol: Do ZERO correlations NEGATE the relationship? *American journal of epidemiology*, *110*(1), 77-87.

72.   Gylling, H., & Simonen, P. (2015). Phytosterols, Phytostanols, and Lipoprotein Metabolism. *Nutrients*, *7*(9), 7965–7977. http://doi.org/10.3390/nu7095374

73.   Sanders TA, Roshanai F. Platelet phospholipid fatty acid composition and function in vegans compared with age- and sex-matched omnivore controls. *Eur J Clin Nutr*. 1992 Nov;46(11):823-31. PubMed PMID: 1425536.

74.   O'Keefe JH Jr, Cordain L, Harris WH, Moe RM, Vogel R. Optimal low-density lipoprotein is 50 to 70 mg/dl: lower is better and physiologically normal. *J Am Coll Cardiol*. 2004 Jun 2;43(11):2142-6. Review. PubMed PMID: 15172426.

75.   McDougall, Dr. John. "Extreme Nutrition: The Diet of Eskimos." *Dr. McDougall*. April 2015. Web.

76.   Thompson RC, Allam AH, Lombardi GP, Wann LS, Sutherland ML, Sutherland JD, Soliman MA, Frohlich B, Mininberg DT, Monge JM,

Vallodolid CM, Cox SL, Abd el-Maksoud G, Badr I, Miyamoto MI, el-Halim Nur el-Din A, Narula J, Finch CE, Thomas GS. Atherosclerosis across 4000 years of human history: the Horus study of four ancient populations. *Lancet*. 2013 Apr 6;381(9873):1211-22. doi: 10.1016/S0140-6736(13)60598-X. Epub 2013 Mar 12. PubMed PMID: 23489753.

77. Spicer, Jonathan. "Inuit lifespan stagnates while Canada's rises." Reuters. January 23, 2008. Web.

78. Peters PA. An age- and cause decomposition of differences in life expectancy between residents of Inuit Nunangat and residents of the rest of Canada, 1989 to 2008. *Health Rep*. 2013 Dec;24(12):3-9. PubMed PMID: 24363060.

79. Mazess RB, Mather W. Bone mineral content of North Alaskan Eskimos. *Am J Clin Nutr*. 1974 Sep;27(9):916-25. PubMed PMID: 4412233.

80. Møller LN, Koch A, Petersen E, Hjuler T, Kapel CM, Andersen A, Melbye M. Trichinella infection in a hunting community in East Greenland. *Epidemiol Infect*. 2010 Sep;138(9):1252-6. doi: 10.1017/S0950268810000282. Epub 2010 Feb 10. PubMed PMID: 20144253.

81. "Toxic Contamination of the Arctic." *Blue Voice*. 2007. Web.

82. Nowaczyk MJ, Waye JS, Douketis JD. DHCR7 mutation carrier rates and prevalence of the RSH/Smith-Lemli-Opitz syndrome: where are the

patients? *Am J Med Genet A*. 2006 Oct 1;140(19):2057-62. Review. PubMed PMID: 16906538.

83. Svoboda, M. D., Christie, J. M., Eroglu, Y., Freeman, K. A., & Steiner, R. D. (2012). Treatment of Smith-Lemli-Opitz Syndrome and Other Sterol Disorders. *American Journal of Medical Genetics. Part C, Seminars in Medical Genetics*, 0(4), 285–294. http://doi.org/10.1002/ajmg.c.31347

84. Porter FD. Smith-Lemli-Opitz syndrome: pathogenesis, diagnosis and management. *Eur J Hum Genet*. 2008 May;16(5):535-41. doi: 10.1038/ejhg.2008.10. Epub 2008 Feb 20. Review. PubMed PMID: 18285838.

85. Irons MB. Cholesterol in childhood: friend or foe?: Commentary on the article by Merkens et al. on page 726. *Pediatr Res*. 2004 Nov;56(5):679-81. Review. PubMed PMID: 15496612.

86. Steinberg, D., Grundy, S. M., Mok, H. Y. I., Turner, J. D., Weinstein, D. B., Brown, W. V., & Albers, J. J. (1979). Metabolic Studies in an Unusual Case of Asymptomatic Familial Hypobetalipoproteinemia with Hypoalphalipoproteinemia and Fasting Chylomicronemia. *Journal of Clinical Investigation*, 64(1), 292–301.

87. "About Cholesterol." *American Heart Association*. April 2017. Web.

88. Mills, Dr. Milton R. "The Comparative Anatomy of Eating." Web.

89.   Bluejay, Michael. "Humans Are Naturally Plant-Eaters." Michael Bluejay: Vegetarian Guide. December 2015. Web.

90.   Spitze AR, Wong DL, Rogers QR, Fascetti AJ. Taurine concentrations in animal feed ingredients; cooking influences taurine content. *J Anim Physiol Anim Nutr (Berl)*. 2003 Aug;87(7-8):251-62. PubMed PMID: 12864905.

91.   Bodie J, Lewis J, Schow D, Monga M. Laboratory evaluations of erectile dysfunction: an evidence based approach. *J Urol.* 2003 Jun;169(6):2262-4. PubMed

92.   Walczak MK, Lokhandwala N, Hodge MB, Guay AT. Prevalence of cardiovascular risk factors in erectile dysfunction. *J Gend Specif Med.* 2002 Nov-Dec;5(6):19-24. PubMed PMID: 12503222.

93.   Dolkas L, Stanley C, Smith AM, Vilke GM. Deaths associated with choking in San Diego County. *J Forensic Sci.* 2007 Jan;52(1):176-9. PubMed PMID: 17209932.

94.   Cartmill M. Rethinking primate origins. *Science.* 1974 Apr 26;184(4135):436-43.PubMed PMID: 4819676.

95.   "First Primates: Meet Your Ancestors." Science Now. July 2008. Web.

96.   Barton, R. A. (2004). Binocularity and brain evolution in primates. *Proceedings of the National Academy of Sciences of the United States of America,* *101*(27), 10113–10115. http://doi.org/10.1073/pnas.0401955101

97. Changizi MA, Shimojo S. "X-ray vision" and the evolution of forward-facing eyes. *J Theor Biol.* 2008 Oct 21;254(4):756-67. doi: 10.1016/j.jtbi.2008.07.011. Epub 2008 Jul 15. PubMed PMID: 18682253.

98. Melin AD, Young HC, Mosdossy KN, Fedigan LM. Seasonality, extractive foraging and the evolution of primate sensorimotor intelligence. *J Hum Evol.* 2014 Jun;71:77-86. doi: 10.1016/j.jhevol.2014.02.009. Epub 2014 Mar 15. PubMed PMID: 24636732.

99. Adler, Jerry. "Why Fire Makes Us Human." *Smithsonian Magazine.* June 2013. Web.

100. Milton K. Nutritional characteristics of wild primate foods: do the diets of our closest living relatives have lessons for us? *Nutrition.* 1999 Jun;15(6):488-98. Review. PubMed PMID: 10378206.

101. Clarke, R., Frost, C., Collins, R., Appleby, P., & Peto, R. (1997). Dietary lipids and blood cholesterol: quantitative meta-analysis of metabolic ward studies. *BMJ : British Medical Journal, 314*(7074), 112–117.

102. Kitahara CM, Berrington de González A, Freedman ND, Huxley R, Mok Y, Jee SH, Samet JM. Total cholesterol and cancer risk in a large prospective study in Korea. *J Clin Oncol.* 2011 Apr 20;29(12):1592-8. doi: 10.1200/JCO.2010.31.5200. Epub 2011 Mar 21. PubMed PMID: 21422422; PubMed Central PMCID: PMC3082977.

103. Danilo C, Frank PG. Cholesterol and breast cancer development. *Curr Opin Pharmacol.* 2012 Dec;12(6):677-82. doi: 10.1016/j.coph.2012.07.009. Epub 2012 Aug 3. Review. PubMed PMID: 22867847.

104. Li YC, Park MJ, Ye SK, Kim CW, Kim YN. Elevated levels of cholesterol-rich lipid rafts in cancer cells are correlated with apoptosis sensitivity induced by cholesterol-depleting agents. *Am J Pathol.* 2006 Apr;168(4):1107-18; quiz 1404-5. PubMed PMID: 16565487; PubMed Central PMCID: PMC1606567.

105. de la Torre JC. Alzheimer disease as a vascular disorder: nosological evidence. *Stroke.* 2002 Apr;33(4):1152-62. Review. PubMed PMID: 11935076.

106. Benjamin, M. M., & Roberts, W. C. (2013). Facts and principles learned at the 39th Annual Williamsburg Conference on Heart Disease. *Proceedings (Baylor University. Medical Center), 26*(2), 124–136.

107. Roberts, W. C. (2007). Facts and ideas from anywhere. *Proceedings (Baylor University. Medical Center), 20*(2), 200–208.

108. Le LT, Sabaté J. Beyond meatless, the health effects of vegan diets: findings from the Adventist cohorts. *Nutrients.* 2014 May 27;6(6):2131-47. doi: 10.3390/nu6062131. Review. PubMed PMID: 24871675; PubMed Central PMCID: PMC4073139.

109. Tantamango-Bartley, Y., Jaceldo-Siegl, K., Fan, J., & Fraser, G. (2013). VEGETARIAN DIETS AND THE INCIDENCE OF CANCER IN A LOW-RISK POPULATION. *Cancer Epidemiology, Biomarkers & Prevention : A Publication of the American Association for Cancer Research, Cosponsored by the American Society of Preventive Oncology, 22*(2), 286–294. http://doi.org/10.1158/1055-9965.EPI-12-1060

110. Pan, A., Sun, Q., Bernstein, A. M., Schulze, M. B., Manson, J. E., Stampfer, M. J., … Hu, F. B. (2012). Red Meat Consumption and Mortality: Results from Two Prospective Cohort Studies. *Archives of Internal Medicine, 172*(7), 555–563. http://doi.org/10.1001/archinternmed.2011.2287

111. "Vitamin A." *National Institutes of Health*. March 2, 2018. Web.

112. Tang G. Bioconversion of dietary provitamin A carotenoids to vitamin A in humans. *Am J Clin Nutr*. 2010 May;91(5):1468S-1473S. doi: 10.3945/ajcn.2010.28674G. Epub 2010 Mar 3. PubMed PMID: 20200262; PubMed Central PMCID: PMC2854912.

113. Penniston KL, Tanumihardjo SA. The acute and chronic toxic effects of vitamin A. *Am J Clin Nutr*. 2006 Feb;83(2):191-201. Review. PubMed PMID: 16469975.

114. Schüpbach R, Wegmüller R, Berguerand C, Bui M, Herter-Aeberli I. Micronutrient status and intake in omnivores, vegetarians and vegans in

Switzerland. *Eur J Nutr.* 2017 Feb;56(1):283-293. doi: 10.1007/s00394-015-1079-7. Epub 2015 Oct 26. PubMed PMID: 26502280.

115. "Vitamin B12." *National Institutes of Health.* March 2, 2018. Web.

116. Schneider, Zenon and Stroiński, Andrzej . *Comprehensive B12: Chemistry, Biochemistry, Nutrition, Ecology, Medicine.* New York: Walter de Gruyter, 1987. Print.

117. Martens JH, Barg H, Warren MJ, Jahn D. Microbial production of vitamin B12. Appl Microbiol Biotechnol. 2002 Mar;58(3):275-85. Epub 2001 Dec 20. Review. PubMed PMID: 11935176.

118. Watanabe, F., Yabuta, Y., Bito, T., & Teng, F. (2014). Vitamin B_{12}-Containing Plant Food Sources for Vegetarians. *Nutrients, 6*(5), 1861–1873. http://doi.org/10.3390/nu6051861

119. Weber MF, Verhoeff J, Holzhauer M, Bartels CJ, van Wuijckhuise L, Vellema P. [Vitamin B12 supplementation and milk production on farms with 'chronic wasting' cattle]. *Tijdschr Diergeneeskd.* 2001 Mar 15;126(6):218-23. Dutch. PubMed PMID: 11285643.

120. Saunders AV, Craig WJ, Baines SK, Posen JS. Iron and vegetarian diets. *Med J Aust.* 2013 Aug 19;199(4 Suppl):S11-6. PubMed PMID: 25369923.

121. "Vitamin D." *National Institutes of Health.* March 2, 2018. Web.

122. Forrest KY, Stuhldreher WL. Prevalence and correlates of vitamin D deficiency in US adults. *Nutr Res.* 2011 Jan;31(1):48-54. doi: 10.1016/j.nutres.2010.12.001. PubMed PMID: 21310306.

123. Palmer, Ashley. "2011 Vegetarian and Vegan Stats." *PETA.* 2011. Web.

124. Nair, R., & Maseeh, A. (2012). Vitamin D: The "sunshine" vitamin. *Journal of Pharmacology & Pharmacotherapeutics, 3*(2), 118–126. http://doi.org/10.4103/0976-500X.95506

125. "Omega-3 Fatty Acids." *National Institutes of Health.* March 2, 2018. Web.

126. Sanders TA. DHA status of vegetarians. *Prostaglandins Leukot Essent Fatty Acids.* 2009 Aug-Sep;81(2-3):137-41. doi: 10.1016/j.plefa.2009.05.013. Epub 2009 Jun 4. Review. PubMed PMID: 19500961.

127. Welch, Ailsa & A Bingham, S & T Khaw, K. (2008). Estimated conversion of -linolenic acid to long chain n-3 polyunsaturated fatty acids is greater than expected in non fish-eating vegetarians and non fish-eating meat-eaters than in fish-eaters. *Journal of human nutrition and dietetics : the official journal of the British Dietetic Association.* 21. 404. 10.1111/j.1365-277X.2008.00881_43.x.

128. Gerster H. Can adults adequately convert alpha-linolenic acid (18:3n-3) to eicosapentaenoic acid (20:5n-3) and docosahexaenoic acid (22:6n-3)? *Int J Vitam Nutr Res.* 1998;68(3):159-73. Review. PubMed PMID: 9637947.

129. Oken E, Choi AL, Karagas MR, Mariën K, Rheinberger CM, Schoeny R, Sunderland E, Korrick S. Which fish should I eat? Perspectives influencing

fish consumption choices. *Environ Health Perspect.* 2012 Jun;120(6):790-8. doi: 10.1289/ehp.1104500. Epub 2012 Feb 22. Review. PubMed PMID: 22534056; PubMed Central PMCID: PMC3385441.

130. Bao Y, Han J, Hu FB, Giovannucci EL, Stampfer MJ, Willett WC, Fuchs CS. Association of nut consumption with total and cause-specific mortality. *N Engl J Med.* 2013 Nov 21;369(21):2001-11. doi: 10.1056/NEJMoa1307352. PubMed PMID: 24256379; PubMed Central PMCID: PMC3931001.

131. Rizos EC, Ntzani EE, Bika E, Kostapanos MS, Elisaf MS. Association between omega-3 fatty acid supplementation and risk of major cardiovascular disease events: a systematic review and meta-analysis. *JAMA.* 2012 Sep 12;308(10):1024-33. doi: 10.1001/2012.jama.11374. Review. PubMed PMID: 22968891.

132. "Vitamin K." *National Institutes of Health.* March 2, 2018. Web.

133. Conly JM, Stein K, Worobetz L, Rutledge-Harding S. The contribution of vitamin K2 (menaquinones) produced by the intestinal microflora to human nutritional requirements for vitamin K. *Am J Gastroenterol.* 1994 Jun;89(6):915-23. PubMed PMID: 8198105.

134. Wallin, R., Schurgers, L., & Wajih, N. (2008). Effects of the Blood Coagulation Vitamin K as an Inhibitor of Arterial Calcification. *Thrombosis Research, 122*(3), 411–417. http://doi.org/10.1016/j.thromres.2007.12.005

135. Dow, C. A., Stauffer, B. L., Greiner, J. J., & DeSouza, C. A. (2014). Influence of Dietary Saturated Fat Intake on Endothelial Fibrinolytic Capacity in Adults. *The American Journal of Cardiology, 114*(5), 783–788. http://doi.org/10.1016/j.amjcard.2014.05.066

136. Levy Y, Maor I, Presser D, Aviram M. Consumption of eggs with meals increases the susceptibility of human plasma and low-density lipoprotein to lipid peroxidation. *Ann Nutr Metab.* 1996;40(5):243-51. PubMed PMID: 9001684.

137. Nicholls SJ, Lundman P, Harmer JA, Cutri B, Griffiths KA, Rye KA, Barter PJ, Celermajer DS. Consumption of saturated fat impairs the anti-inflammatory properties of high-density lipoproteins and endothelial function. *J Am Coll Cardiol.* 2006 Aug 15;48(4):715-20. Epub 2006 Jul 24. PubMed PMID: 16904539.

138. Geleijnse JM, Vermeer C, Grobbee DE, Schurgers LJ, Knapen MH, van der Meer IM, Hofman A, Witteman JC. Dietary intake of menaquinone is associated with a reduced risk of coronary heart disease: the Rotterdam Study. *J Nutr.* 2004 Nov;134(11):3100-5. PubMed PMID: 15514282.

139. Nimptsch K, Rohrmann S, Kaaks R, Linseisen J. Dietary vitamin K intake in relation to cancer incidence and mortality: results from the Heidelberg cohort of the European Prospective Investigation into Cancer and

Nutrition (EPIC-Heidelberg). *Am J Clin Nutr.* 2010 May;91(5):1348-58. doi: 10.3945/ajcn.2009.28691. Epub 2010 Mar 24. PubMed PMID: 20335553.

140. Melina V, Craig W, Levin S. Position of the Academy of Nutrition and Dietetics: Vegetarian Diets. *J Acad Nutr Diet.* 2016 Dec;116(12):1970-1980. doi: 10.1016/j.jand.2016.09.025. PubMed PMID: 27886704.

141. Allen NE, Appleby PN, Davey GK, Kaaks R, Rinaldi S, Key TJ. The associations of diet with serum insulin-like growth factor I and its main binding proteins in 292 women meat-eaters, vegetarians, and vegans. *Cancer Epidemiol Biomarkers Prev.* 2002 Nov;11(11):1441-8. PubMed PMID: 12433724.

142. Joy JM, Lowery RP, Wilson JM, Purpura M, De Souza EO, Wilson SM, Kalman DS, Dudeck JE, Jäger R. The effects of 8 weeks of whey or rice protein supplementation on body composition and exercise performance. *Nutr J.* 2013 Jun 20;12:86. doi: 10.1186/1475-2891-12-86. PubMed PMID: 23782948; PubMed Central PMCID: PMC3698202.

143. McDougall J. Plant foods have a complete amino acid composition. *Circulation.* 2002 Jun 25;105(25):e197; author reply e197. PubMed PMID: 12082008.

144. Appleby PN, Thorogood M, Mann JI, Key TJ. The Oxford Vegetarian Study: an overview. *Am J Clin Nutr.* 1999 Sep;70(3 Suppl):525S-531S. doi: 10.1093/ajcn/70.3.525s. PubMed PMID: 10479226.

145. Hamilton-Reeves JM, Vazquez G, Duval SJ, Phipps WR, Kurzer MS, Messina MJ. Clinical studies show no effects of soy protein or isoflavones on reproductive hormones in men: results of a meta-analysis. *Fertil Steril.* 2010 Aug;94(3):997-1007. doi: 10.1016/j.fertnstert.2009.04.038. Epub 2009 Jun 12. Review. PubMed PMID: 19524224.

146. Messina M. Soybean isoflavone exposure does not have feminizing effects on men: a critical examination of the clinical evidence. *Fertil Steril.* 2010 May 1;93(7):2095-104. doi: 10.1016/j.fertnstert.2010.03.002. Epub 2010 Apr 8. Review. PubMed PMID: 20378106.

147. Kalman, D., Feldman, S., Martinez, M., Krieger, D. R., & Tallon, M. J. (2007). Effect of protein source and resistance training on body composition and sex hormones. *Journal of the International Society of Sports Nutrition, 4,* 4. http://doi.org/10.1186/1550-2783-4-4

148. Dickson RB, Clark CR. Estrogen receptors in the male. *Arch Androl.* 1981 Nov;7(3):205-17. PubMed PMID: 7305538.

149. McCarty MF. Isoflavones made simple - genistein's agonist activity for the beta-type estrogen receptor mediates their health benefits. *Med Hypotheses.* 2006;66(6):1093-114. Epub 2006 Mar 2. PubMed PMID: 16513288.

150. Chavarro JE, Toth TL, Sadio SM, Hauser R. Soy food and isoflavone intake in relation to semen quality parameters among men from an infertility clinic. *Hum Reprod.* 2008 Nov;23(11):2584-90. doi: 10.1093/humrep/den243.

Epub 2008 Jul 23. PubMed PMID: 18650557; PubMed Central PMCID: PMC2721724.

151. Vandenplas Y, Castrellon PG, Rivas R, Gutiérrez CJ, Garcia LD, Jimenez JE, Anzo A, Hegar B, Alarcon P. Safety of soya-based infant formulas in children. *Br J Nutr.* 2014 Apr 28;111(8):1340-60. doi: 10.1017/S0007114513003942. Epub 2014 Feb 10. Review. PubMed PMID: 24507712.

152. Strom BL, Schinnar R, Ziegler EE, Barnhart KT, Sammel MD, Macones GA, Stallings VA, Drulis JM, Nelson SE, Hanson SA. Exposure to soy-based formula in infancy and endocrinological and reproductive outcomes in young adulthood. *JAMA.* 2001 Aug 15;286(7):807-14. PubMed PMID: 11497534.

153. Vaarala O, Knip M, Paronen J, Hämäläinen AM, Muona P, Väätäinen M, Ilonen J, Simell O, Akerblom HK. Cow's milk formula feeding induces primary immunization to insulin in infants at genetic risk for type 1 diabetes. *Diabetes.* 1999 Jul;48(7):1389-94. PubMed PMID: 10389843.

154. Gottlieb, S. (2000). Early exposure to cows' milk raises risk of diabetes in high risk children. *BMJ : British Medical Journal, 321*(7268), 1040.

155. Karjalainen J, Martin JM, Knip M, Ilonen J, Robinson BH, Savilahti E, Akerblom HK, Dosch HM. A bovine albumin peptide as a possible trigger of insulin-dependent diabetes mellitus. *N Engl J Med.* 1992 Jul

30;327(5):302-7. Erratum in: N Engl J Med 1992 Oct 22;327(17):1252. PubMed PMID: 1377788.

156. Chen M, Rao Y, Zheng Y, Wei S, Li Y, Guo T, Yin P. Association between soy isoflavone intake and breast cancer risk for pre- and post-menopausal women: a meta-analysis of epidemiological studies. *PLoS One*. 2014 Feb 20;9(2):e89288. doi: 10.1371/journal.pone.0089288. eCollection 2014. PubMed PMID: 24586662; PubMed Central PMCID: PMC3930722.

157. Arjmandi BH, Khalil DA, Smith BJ, Lucas EA, Juma S, Payton ME, Wild RA. Soy protein has a greater effect on bone in postmenopausal women not on hormone replacement therapy, as evidenced by reducing bone resorption and urinary calcium excretion. *J Clin Endocrinol Metab*. 2003 Mar;88(3):1048-54. PubMed PMID: 12629084.

158. Kelsey TW, Li LQ, Mitchell RT, Whelan A, Anderson RA, Wallace WH. A validated age-related normative model for male total testosterone shows increasing variance but no decline after age 40 years. *PLoS One*. 2014 Oct 8;9(10):e109346. doi: 10.1371/journal.pone.0109346. eCollection 2014. Erratum in: PLoS One. 2015;10(2):e0117674. PubMed PMID: 25295520; PubMed Central PMCID: PMC4190174.

159. Fui, M. N. T., Dupuis, P., & Grossmann, M. (2014). Lowered testosterone in male obesity: mechanisms, morbidity and management. *Asian Journal of Andrology*, *16*(2), 223–231. http://doi.org/10.4103/1008-682X.122365

160. Meikle AW, Stringham JD, Woodward MG, McMurry MP. Effects of a fat-containing meal on sex hormones in men. *Metabolism*. 1990 Sep;39(9):943-6. PubMed PMID: 2392062.

161. Fryar, Cheryl D et al. "Prevalence of Overweight, Obesity, and Extreme Obesity Among Adults: United States, 1960–1962 Through 2011–2012." *Centers for Disease Control and Prevention*. November 6, 2015. Web.

162. Maruyama K, Oshima T, Ohyama K. Exposure to exogenous estrogen through intake of commercial milk produced from pregnant cows. *Pediatr Int*. 2010 Feb;52(1):33-8. doi: 10.1111/j.1442-200X.2009.02890.x. Epub 2009 May 22. PubMed PMID: 19496976.

163. Possemiers S, Heyerick A, Robbens V, De Keukeleire D, Verstraete W. Activation of proestrogens from hops (Humulus lupulus L.) by intestinal microbiota; conversion of isoxanthohumol into 8-prenylnaringenin. *J Agric Food Chem*. 2005 Aug 10;53(16):6281-8. PubMed PMID: 16076107.

164. Schaefer O, Hümpel M, Fritzemeier KH, Bohlmann R, Schleuning WD. 8-Prenyl naringenin is a potent ERalpha selective phytoestrogen present in hops and beer. *J Steroid Biochem Mol Biol*. 2003 Feb;84(2-3):359-60. PubMed PMID: 12711023.

165. Ellingboe J, Varanelli CC. Ethanol inhibits testosterone biosynthesis by direct action on Leydig cells. *Res Commun Chem Pathol Pharmacol*. 1979 Apr;24(1):87-102. PubMed PMID: 219455.

166. Logan BK, Distefano S. Ethanol content of various foods and soft drinks and their potential for interference with a breath-alcohol test. *J Anal Toxicol.* 1998 May-Jun;22(3):181-3. PubMed PMID: 9602932.

167. van Thiel DH, Gavaler JS, Cobb CF, Sherins RJ, Lester R. Alcohol-induced testicular atrophy in the adult male rat. *Endocrinology.* 1979 Oct;105(4):888-95. PubMed PMID: 477602.

168. Van Thiel, D. H. (1979). Feminization of chronic alcoholic men: a formulation. *The Yale Journal of Biology and Medicine, 52*(2), 219–225.

169. Galvão-Teles A, Gonçalves L, Carvalho H, Monteiro E. Alterations of testicular morphology in alcoholic disease. Alcohol Clin Exp Res. 1983 Spring;7(2):144-9. Review. PubMed PMID: 6346916.

170. *Alcohol Clin Exp Res.* 1983 Spring;7(2):131-248. Review.

171. Islam MN, Khalil MI, Islam MA, Gan SH. Toxic compounds in honey. *J Appl Toxicol.* 2014 Jul;34(7):733-42. doi: 10.1002/jat.2952. Epub 2013 Nov 11. Review. PubMed PMID: 24214851.

172. Fry, T. C. "Article #1: Why Honey is a Harmful Food." *Raw Food Explained.* 2006. Web.

173. Watanabe, M. (1994). Pollination worries rise as honey bees decline. *Science, 265,* 1170.

174. Shimanuki, H. et al. (Research Leader, Bee Research Laboratory, USDA) (1992). Diseases and Pests of Honey Bees. *The Hive and the honey bee.* J. Graham (ed). Hamilton, IL: Dadant.

175. Sugden, E. (Tura-Lura Apiaries) (1996). In Andrew Matheson et al. (eds.), *The Conservation of Bees.* New York: Academic Press.

176. Schmidt, J. & Buchmann, S. (Research Entomologists, Carl Hayden Bee Research Center). (1992). Other Products of the Hive. *The Hive and the honey bee.* J. Graham (ed). Hamilton, IL: Dadant.

177. O'Toole, C. (Hope Entomological Collections, University Museum, Oxford) (1993). Diversity of Native Bees and Agroecosystems. *Hymenoptera and Biodiversity.* J. LaSalle & I.D. Gauld (eds). C.A.B International.

178. Adee, R. (President, American Honey Producers Association) (1992, July 30). *Review of the U.S. Honey Program.* Y4.AG 8/1:102-90.

179. Landgraf, T., Rojas, R., Nguyen, H., Kriegel, F., & Stettin, K. (2011). Analysis of the Waggle Dance Motion of Honeybees for the Design of a Biomimetic Honeybee Robot. *PLoS ONE*, 6(8), e21354. http://doi.org/10.1371/journal.pone.0021354

180. Everding, Gerry. "Insect diet helped early humans build bigger brains, study suggests." *Washington University in St. Louis.* June 25, 2014. Web.

181. Worrall, Simon. "Yes, Animals Think And Feel. Here's How We Know." *National Geographic.* July 15, 2015. Web.

182. Hoole, Jan. "Animals do have feelings – and here's the science to prove it."

iNews. November 29, 2017. Web.

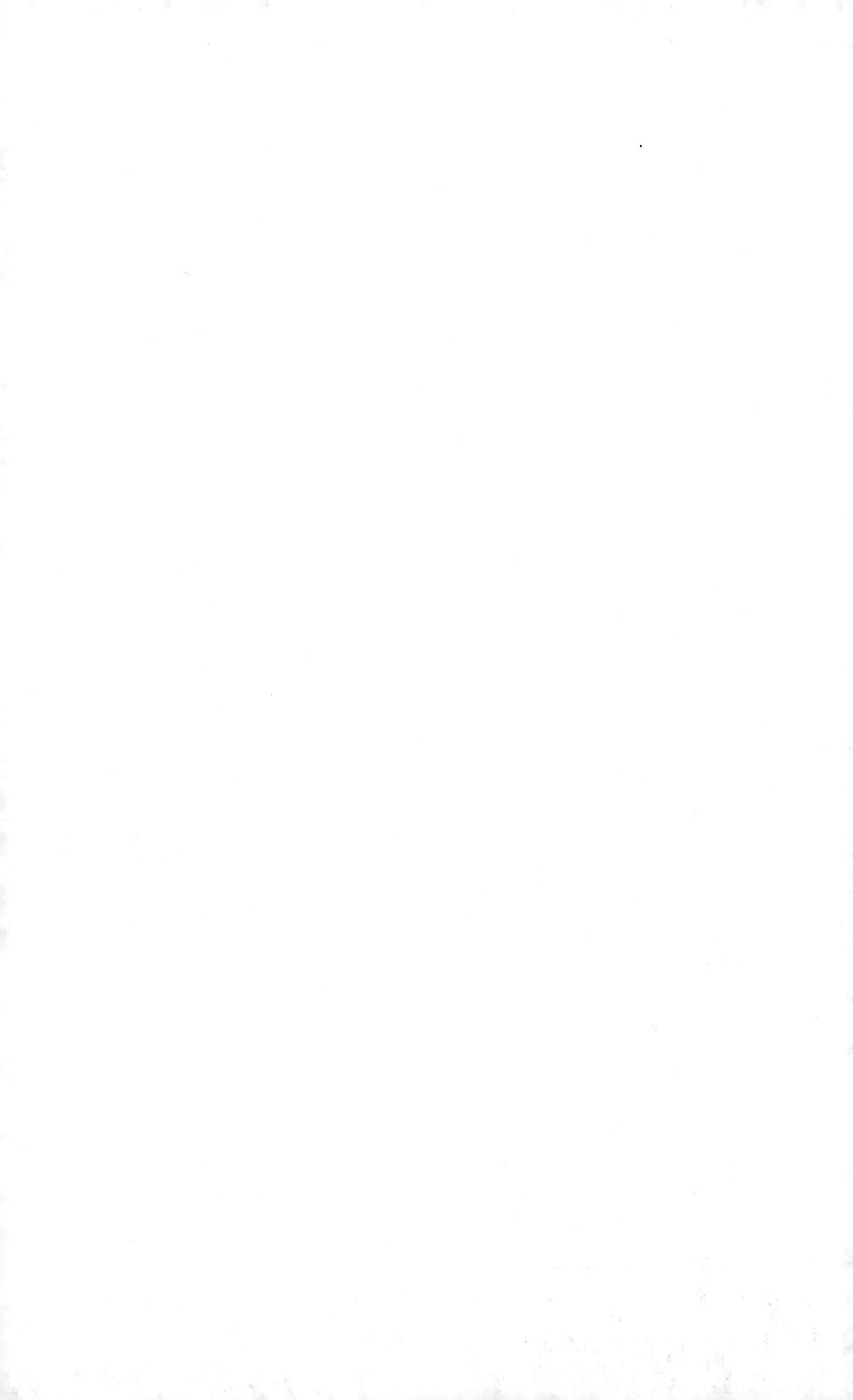